DATE DUE

JUN 1 2 2019			
APR 0 6 2020			

Demco, Inc. 38-293

Living with Insomnia

MCFARLAND HEALTH TOPICS SERIES

Living with Insomnia

*A Guide to Causes, Effects
and Management,
with Personal Accounts*

Phyllis L. Brodsky *and*
Allen Brodsky

Foreword by David N. Neubauer

McFarland Health Topics Series
Elaine A. Moore, *Series Editor*

McFarland & Company, Inc., Publishers
Jefferson, North Carolina, and London

ALSO BY PHYLLIS L. BRODSKY
AND FROM MCFARLAND

*The Control of Childbirth: Women Versus
Medicine Through the Ages* (2008)

LIBRARY OF CONGRESS CATALOGUING-IN-PUBLICATION DATA

Brodsky, Phyllis L., 1936–
   Living with insomnia : a guide to causes, effects and management,
with personal accounts / Phyllis L. Brodsky and Allen Brodsky ;
foreword by David N. Neubauer.
      p.   cm.—(McFarland health topics series)
   [Elaine A. Moore, series editor]
   Includes bibliographical references and index.

   ISBN 978-0-7864-5971-1
   softcover : 50# alkaline paper ∞

   1. Insomnia.   2. Insomniacs—Life skill guides.   I. Brodsky,
Allen.   II. Title.
   RC548.B76   2011
   616.8'4982—dc22   2011003425

BRITISH LIBRARY CATALOGUING DATA ARE AVAILABLE

Front cover images © 2011 Shutterstock

Manufactured in the United States of America

McFarland & Company, Inc., Publishers
   Box 611, Jefferson, North Carolina 28640
   www.mcfarlandpub.com

Acknowledgments

Sharon Dlubala, proprietor of A Novel Idea bookstore in Berlin, Maryland, has been very helpful in searching for books and in recommending books for our project. She has also been timely in supplying the books we purchased for use in our writing and for our permanent library on insomnia. Jim Adcock responded quickly with his outstanding artistic skills each time an exhibit was requested, and again when revisions were desired. The staff at Copy Central, and the proprietress Linda Dearing, also provided ready assistance with many of our printing and formatting needs; we especially mention the skills of Pat Quade in dealing with the many glitches we have had with Word software and computer problems. People like Pat are particularly valuable at moments when someone with little hair is ready to tear out the rest.

We are also grateful to Dr. David N. Neubauer, associate professor on the faculty of the Department of Psychiatry at the Johns Hopkins Medical Institutions, and associate director of their sleep clinic. He kindly provided encouragement for our project, and responded to our tardy request to provide review and comments at a late stage of our writing, only a couple of weeks before our final manuscript was due at McFarland.

Many in our family provided encouragement and suggestions in the initial stages of our proposal and writing, especially John Berry and Rick Kowaleski, who provided comments on our Sleep Questionnaire and other aspects of our project that helped launch our efforts. Friends of the family, grandchildren and many others volunteered to fill out the questionnaires from which the sample narratives in this book were obtained.

Last but not least, we are grateful to each other for patiently considering, again and again and again, the idiosyncratic opinions of each other about what should be in the book, and what should not be in the book, without raising tempers and voices to the point of all-out war. When we submitted the final manuscript to the publisher, we made an agreement to trust their knowledge and not further tinker with the content. In this way, we have saved our marriage and hope that our book will relieve any further insomnia of our own, as well as that of others.

Contents

Foreword

by David N. Neubauer, MD

A good night's sleep is something we tend to take for granted until it eludes us. Without good sleep most of us feel miserable the next day. Many different things potentially can interfere with our ability to sleep well. Sometimes circumstances prevent us from spending sufficient time in bed to get enough sleep, but other times we may be in bed intending to sleep and it just doesn't happen. When frustrating sleeplessness persists and subsequently affects how we feel and function during the daytime, the problem may be insomnia. We all occasionally have a sleepless night. It is no surprise that insomnia is the most common type of sleep disorder. Although insomnia typically has a short duration, for some individuals it may continue for months and years. People suffering with insomnia frequently feel fatigued and complain of poor concentration and memory. They may also feel depressed and irritable. They tend to worry more and more about their inability to sleep well to the point that the worrying perpetuates the insomnia they are worrying about!

Much has been published about the causes, consequences, and treatments of insomnia. Among these are scores of scholarly textbooks, thousands of scientific articles, and innumerable self-help books for the general public. With this book, *Living with Insomnia*, Phyllis and Allen Brodsky provide a welcome addition to the insomnia literature. They offer an overview of normal sleep and discuss the many ways that sleep can be disrupted. The book also gives a sense of how sleep problems can affect the lives of ordinary people. It is most evident in the Brodskys' descriptions of their own sleep, but the many case examples included in the book highlight the wide diversity of sleep patterns and sleep disorders present in the general population. It is

1

especially interesting to see how people vary in the degree to which they regard sleep disturbances as serious problems. Some individuals seek solutions with home remedies or by consulting with doctors, while others try to ignore the nighttime sleep disturbance and somehow muddle along day after day.

I see many patients with the types of sleep difficulties described by the Brodskys in this book. In some cases the causes and solutions are relatively simple. It may be that the person needs to cut back on caffeine, use CPAP for sleep apnea, be treated for a depressed mood, or stop working the night shift. For others the causes may be less evident and the treatment more complex, perhaps involving behavioral therapies, medications, or a combination of both.

I hope that readers of *Living with Insomnia* will reflect more on their sleep and that of their family members and friends who may be suffering from insomnia or other sleep disorders. The science of sleep is growing rapidly and the field of sleep medicine is expanding. Most people will benefit from improvements in their sleep habits and healthy lifestyle routines, but others may need evaluation by a primary care provider or sleep disorders specialist. The important lesson in this book is that life with insomnia does not necessarily mean continuous misery. Rather, insomnia should stimulate an exploration of the factors that are undermining good quality sleep, motivate people toward improved health habits, and encourage them to seek help in finding effective solutions. Good sleep should be valued along with diet and exercise in contributing to our overall physical and mental health.

Dr. Neubauer is an associate professor in the Department of Psychiatry at Johns Hopkins University and is associate director of the university's Sleep Disorders Center. He has specialized in the clinical evaluation and management of patients with sleep disorders for the past 25 years.

Preface

We've all been there. Sleepiness and sluggishness during the day. General tiredness. Irritability. Problems focusing or concentrating on tasks at work or at home. All because we can't sleep, or when we are able to sleep, we wake up feeling just as tired as when we went to bed.

Insomnia is a sleep disorder characterized by difficulty falling asleep or staying asleep, or both. It affects our moods, our productivity, our interactions with others, our physical and mental health—virtually all aspects of our lives—but it doesn't have to be a problem.

We have experienced sleepless nights and subsequent lethargies throughout busy professional careers, and we realized, as longtime authors, that the writers of any book usually learn more new information of personal value to themselves while sharing what they have learned with others. Therefore, we decided to work together on this book, for our own benefit as well as for others.

In searching for information on this subject, we soon found that there were hundreds of books and articles already written on insomnia and other sleep disorders. This was not completely unexpected. However, in examining some books on the subject, we became concerned about the difficult jobs of researching and analyzing the available information. We thought, "How in the world can we do justice to this subject?" But we put our heads together and started thinking. The idea for a useful approach came to us, and we decided to forge ahead.

We thought, because the research and analysis were so overwhelming, and so much of it inaccessible and incomprehensible to the average reader, that what was most likely needed was a condensed review of insomnia so that we all could benefit from the current knowledge of causes, effects and treatments for insomnia and related disorders that take an aggravating and potentially dangers toll on our lives. We thus decided to continue with a book in which we would gather a number of stories from people in our own social and professional communities and include a sample of those stories in our book. We would describe our composite observations and compare them with the most recent findings in authoritative works by insomnia and other sleep disorder experts. In this way, we could provide a general overview of a subject of real importance to many people.

Introduction

The aim of this book is to provide those with sleep problems or chronic insomnia a concise overview of present knowledge of the causes, effects, and possible treatments that could help improve their lives. To this end, the book includes summaries of current knowledge about insomnia and sleep issues taken from research reported in books and articles, with the addition of a limited sample of stories of human interest and information culled from questionnaires and interviews of friends and associates. In this way, we are able to compare, in an easily read publication, current scientific and medical knowledge about insomnia with some real life stories of persons living with insomnia. We believe and hope that these stories, analyses and conclusions will then help many readers improve their sleep habits and lives.

The first two chapters summarize from recent publications the current knowledge of the nature of insomnia, its prevalence, classifications and consequences, and normal sleep patterns and requirements for healthy living. Chapter 3 then "takes a breath" and provides, with some humor, the human interest stories about the authors' personal experiences living with insomnia, and how these experiences relate to the information culled from the first two chapters.

Chapter 4 covers how sleep patterns change with age, so that readers might be able to assist those younger or older in their families, as well as themselves. Chapter 5 provides an overview of sleep disorders and their underlying pathologies that require treatment to overcome difficulties with insomnia. Chapter 6 relates a number of stories from persons interviewed about how they have lived with insomnia, and any suggestions about how they have dealt with or alleviated their problems. The stories presented have been selected to be those that might illustrate a reasonable sample of scenarios of those living with insomnia. Chapter 7 describes some unusual but peculiar effects of disturbed sleep patterns and probable causes, such as sleep walking and night terrors.

Chapter 8 then presents the negative consequences of insomnia and sleep disorders in daily living, health effects, and risks of injuries. Chapter 9 covers treatments that can manage or improve sleep patterns and alleviate the negative consequences.

Chapter 10 provides summaries of the causes, effects, treatments, and any cures, culled from the authors' questionnaires and interviews, compares these findings for consistencies with literature knowledge, and examines any statistically different or apparently new information obtained from the sample of persons living with insomnia. Chapter 11 provides a brief summary and listing of conclusions useful to anyone living with insomnia, as derived from the various aspects of insomnia presented in the previous chapters.

CHAPTER 1

What Is Insomnia?

It seems that almost every morning when I (Phyllis) wake up from a night's sleep (sometimes it is good and sometimes not so good), the first thing I hear from my husband (if he's still in bed and awake) is a report of his night's sleep. Then I give him my report. This ritual gets old after awhile. But sleep seems to rule our lives. It seems it rules other people's lives as well. After reading this book, you will realize you are not alone and there is help for you troubled sleepers. As a reward for writing this book, we are sleeping better.

If I don't get enough sleep at night, I'm not a happy person. I'm tired, irritable, and cranky. Fortunately, for the senior citizen that I am, I'm healthy, active, and do not have any health problems, other than insomnia. Lack of sleep is daunting. I've been troubled by bouts of insomnia for much of my adult life. My problem is exacerbated when I sleep in homes other than my own (such as visiting family and friends) and in hotel rooms. I am particularly troubled when I travel to faraway places by air that cross several time zones.

On the other hand, when Allen loses sleep, because of either poor sleep practices on some nights or waking up thinking of many concerns and not falling back to sleep, he does not worry about it but tries to do his best the following day to pursue his planned work or recreational activities. At this later stage of his life, Allen does not have insomnia, but at some earlier stages, as described in Chapter 3, Allen "lived with" insomnia.

Neubauer has discussed the difficulties in defining insomnia, the range of definitions employed by professionals, and the need for specific definitions in standardized medical coding in order to carry on sleep research. After describing some of the difficulties, one simple way that Neubauer concludes that he can define insomnia is:

"Fundamentally, 'I have insomnia' means (1) 'I can't sleep' and (2) 'I'm suffering.'"[1] This indicates his opinion that a person must have a serious problem with his sleep habits to be considered an insomniac. From the more complete descriptions of our sleep habits in Chapter 3, one might conclude that I (Phyllis) (perceptions 1 and 2 together) now have a problem with insomnia, whereas Allen (usually perception 1 alone on occasion) does not. However, in Allen's own description in Chapter 3 of his sleep habits throughout life, it is apparent that during times of stress, Allen did suffer from "short-term" insomnia, as defined later in this chapter.

In Chapter 6, we will see some of the difficulties of placing a person in a category of insomnia. In placing persons in insomnia categories, considerable judgment was needed to weighing frequency and severity of sleep problems. Sometimes a person in our sample would indicate problems sleeping only a fraction of the days in a month, and was satisfied with sleep habits the rest of the month. However, when someone had problems only a fraction of the month, but these sleep problems caused only temporary, but serious, disturbances in either the person's work or homelife, then if the problems seemed serious enough, the person was placed in either the category of living with insomnia or the more serious category, depending on our judgment of seriousness. Also, the four perspectives used by Neubauer in diagnosing insomnia were found to come into play when in Chapter 6 we were placing men and women into categories, after writing the narratives from their sleep questionnaires: diseases—how seriously they influenced sleep; measurements—amounts and timing of sleep stages relative to their life requirements; behaviors—their attitudes, expectations for sleep, and degree of worry over sleep loss; and lifestyles—the effects of their sleep loss on their livelihood and general lifestyles.

I (Phyllis), in writing the early part of this book, will now introduce the concepts of insomnia with just some brief personal examples.

On a recent trip to Israel (10 hours going and 13 hours returning), I suffered severe jet lag. Between the cramped seating, the need to frequently find more comfortable positions, the chilly draft, and often too much light, I suffered with little rest—not too silently—throughout the flight. Allen was very patient with me, especially since my feet were somewhere on his lap most of the time. I did not feel great upon arriving in Israel.

I must admit that I took a nightly sleeping pill for half of the ten days we were on this trip, which helped. I wanted to be alert and enjoy, which I did immensely. It was a wonderful tour. Ten days later, we returned to the States in a 13-hour flight crossing six time zones. Once we returned home (westward bound), I again had trouble sleeping through the night. The worst of it was waking up at three or four in the morning, wide eyed and alert, for almost a month. I wasn't alone, however. While complaining to friends who were on this trip (we were a group of 22 and knew each other), they were experiencing similar sleep disturbances.

With the help of sleep aids, I eventually returned to my usual sleep patterns, although my "usual" was not great to begin with. There is a physiologic reason for jet lag that we'll explain in the next chapter in discussing biological clocks, circadian rhythms, and normal sleep. I've had chronic insomnia for so many years that I cannot remember when it started. This affliction has always been disturbing to me. But I am not alone; many people suffer from some form of insomnia.

I take aerobic classes several times a week at a nearby gym. Most people taking these classes (including myself) arrive five to ten minutes before the class begins. Because most of these people are women, we chat. Some of the things we chat about are our sleep. So, I knew I was not alone in dealing with sleep issues, even before starting work on this book.

I'll tell more of my story in Chapter 3. My husband, Allen, will also tell his story. We will also tell the personal stories of others in Chapter 6 to give typical perspectives of what insomnia is all about, what people do to relieve their sleep problems, and what works and what doesn't work for them.

According to an article appearing in the March 8, 2010, issue of *USA Today*, the National Sleep Foundation (NSF) had just completed its annual "Sleep in America Poll." Findings from this poll revealed how much sleep Americans get, what their bedtime habits are, how many seek medical attention, and how many are taking medication for sleep. The NSF also sought to explore the sleep habits of different ethnic groups. Thomas Balkin, chairman of the foundation's board, said, "Fewer than half—only about four in 10—of respondents from each ethnic group say they get a good night's sleep on most nights." Balkin contends that inadequate sleep is associated with obesity, heart disease, and diabetes.[2]

The intent of this chapter is to define insomnia, since it is the focus of this book. Then we will focus on normal sleep patterns in the next chapter. Other aspects of insomnia and related sleep disorders, underlying pathologies and causes, parasomnias, effects of sleep deprivation, and treatments will also be described in later chapters. In the absence of known causes, underlying sleep disorders, or specific pathologies, the cause of insomnia is unknown. When there is no known cause, it is referred to as primary or idiopathic insomnia.

If anyone were asked to define insomnia, the answer would most likely be, "I have trouble sleeping." They would be correct, but the definition is far more complex. The term "insomnia" can be ambiguous; it is a broad generalization of many sleep disturbances and disorders. It suggests that an individual is not able to sleep, but the term "insomnia" alone does not specify a particular pattern of sleep disturbance. A definition of insomnia is more than just having difficulty getting to sleep or staying asleep; there must also be daytime symptoms, such as complaints of sleepiness or fatigue. To further complicate the picture, insomnia is often a symptom of a specific sleep disorder or underlying medical or psychological problem.

In the absence of known underlying pathologies, insomnias fall into the following categories: (1) difficulty falling asleep (sleep onset problem); (2) falling asleep easily, but waking up during the night and not being able to get back to sleep (sleep maintenance difficulty); and (3) waking up too early in the morning. A person might have a combination of two or all three of these categories.

Insomnia is also classified as transient (or short term), intermittent, or chronic (long term). Transient insomnia lasts a short period of time, usually less than three weeks. If transient insomnia recurs, it is then referred to as intermittent. If the problem recurs frequently for more than a month, then it is considered to be a chronic condition.[3]

Sleep specialists concur that there are many causes of insomnia. Sleep disorders are classified in several ways, specified in two professional manuals. *The Diagnostic and Statistical Manual of Mental Disorders* (DSM-IV) lists underlying mental disorders, medical conditions, and medicinal substances that can cause insomnia. *The International Classification of Sleep Disorders* (ICSD) identifies the many underlying causes of insomnia.[4] These disorders are described in detail in chapters 5 and 7 of our book.

The ICSD states that short-term insomnias are almost universal. It defines short-term insomnia (also referred to as "sub-acute") as sleep problems that last from one week to three months duration. Short-term insomnia is also described as "a complaint of insomnia temporally associated with a reaction to an identifiable stressor," such as anxiety, restlessness, pain, or other physical or psychological symptoms. The definition should also include a complaint of daytime tiredness, dysfunction in the form of change in normal energy level, alertness, cognitive function, or behavioral or emotional state.[5]

Symptoms of insomnia can also be caused by such underlying problems as pain, depression, psychological or psychiatric disorders, heart, lung or kidney diseases, premenstrual syndrome, pregnancy, menopause, apnea, restless leg syndrome, or any number of underlying sleep disorders or parasomnias. Insomnia can also be caused by stress and anxiety, consuming alcohol or caffeinated beverages close to bedtime, jet lag, working night shifts or swing shifts, too much light in the bedroom, and noxious noise (such as your partner snoring).

Alcohol causes a reduced amount of REM sleep, total amount of sleep, and multiple awakenings. Caffeine is a stimulant which disturbs natural sleep and has a long half life — about three to seven hours — so that even if consumed in the afternoon it can disrupt sleep by nighttime. There are other underlying sleep disorders that cause insomnia, which are discussed in succeeding chapters. There may also possibly be a genetic connection.

There are structures located at the base of the brain that secrete various chemicals — called neurohormones — that regulate sleep-wake cycles. There are actually two distinct centers: one is responsible for being awake and the other for allowing us to sleep. Our wakefulness center dominates, being more readily stimulated by external and internal signals. External signals are light, sound, and temperature; internal signals include such musings as anticipation of next day's events, worry, sadness, stress, and physical ailments, such as pain.[6] The fact that the alert center dominates is an evolutionary means of enabling us to wake up in the face of danger to defend and protect ourselves and family from external danger. This is why a mother wakes up easily to the sound of her baby crying (in most instances).

Insomnia is not a normal state; it is a state of imbalance of the two centers, in which the alert center overrides the sleep center. For some reason, in some people, the alert center takes over and dominates for most of the night. However, there are instances when insomnia can be considered, temporarily, a normal state. Such is the case when a special event such as a birthday party or other happy occasion is anticipated. The anticipation of the start of a new job or entrance into a university can override the need to sleep. Also, the emotional response to a tragic event, such as death of a close family member or friend, can cause temporary insomnia. For the person who does not have chronic insomnia, this normal response is generally temporary until the event passes or the stage of grief is resolved. Of course, grief can last a long time for many people.

Insomnia affects people of all ages across the life cycle, but becomes more prevalent as people age. It is also more prevalent in women, particularly during menstruation, childbearing, before, during, and after menopause. The prevalence of insomnia varies greatly depending on the population surveyed or interviewed, and how data is collected and analyzed.

In a 2000 issue of the journal *Sleep*, the authors indicated that the prevalence of insomnias in the United States population is about 35 percent.[7] They explained that many epidemiologic studies are confounded by the methods used in the study, people's descriptions of their sleep disturbances, and other factors.

Dr. David N. Neubauer wrote that, according to the National Sleep Foundation (NSF), dating back to 1999, half of America's adults experience one or more symptoms of insomnia at least a few nights a week.[8] The NSF estimated that 47 million Americans suffer from sleep disorders. In 2003, the National Institute of Health (NIH) estimated 50 to 70 million Americans have sleep-related problems.[9] In his book, *Sleep*, Dr. Carlos Schenck states, "Insomnia, which affects about 58 percent of American adults at some point in their lives, is the most common of all sleep complaints and true sleep problems."[10] Results from a more recent nationwide survey, conducted by the Centers for Disease Control and Prevention (CDC) in 2008, showed that, among 403,981 adult respondents, 11.1 percent reported insufficient sleep every day for the 30 days preceding the survey.[11] Insomnia can be a devastating affliction for some individuals. Michael Jackson had to resort to being given anesthesia by his personal physician. Together, all the sleep medications and the anesthetic led to his untimely death. The consequences of poor sleep can take its toll on many individuals, hopefully not as devastating as Michael Jackson's case.

Chronic insomnia can lead to sleep deprivation. Dr. William C. Dement, who has studied sleep science since 1952, described the dangers of sleep debt in his book, *The Promise of Sleep*. He explained that when a person gets significantly less sleep than he or she requires, which is based upon how he or she feels the next day, the person builds up hours of sleep lost, or sleep debt.[12] The dangerous effects of sleep debt are directly related to the amount of lost sleep. Sleep debt can result from a person's choice to go to sleep late and arise early, existing on substantially less sleep than needed. More of the consequences of sleep loss are covered in Chapter 8.

In general, effects of sleep deprivation are feelings of tiredness, fatigue, or crankiness; and lack of energy and enthusiasm for work, school, or usual daily activities. Falling asleep at work, at meetings, or in the classroom can be embarrassing to the person; he or she misses important information or has other consequences. Severe sleep disturbances can also lead to major medical problems, injuries, and disasters.

Falling asleep at the wheel can be devastating, not only to the insomniac, but to anyone else on the road. In his book, *A Woman's Guide to Sleep Disorders*, Dr. Meir H. Kryger stated, "Every year, sleepy drivers cause an estimated 20 percent of car accidents, as high as 1.2 million crashes, resulting in huge numbers of deaths and injuries and billions in property damage."[13] Loss of sleep can also cause such problems as depression, anxiety, addictions to alcohol and drugs, and physical health problems.

Prior to the invention of the electric light, which can simulate daytime light, people's natural rhythm (biological clock) was in tune with nature's rhythm. When it became dark, people were no longer able to do their chores. In prehistoric times it was dangerous to roam around at night. Instead of successfully hunting for food, hunters could themselves become prey. The invention of oil lamps allowed people to extend their day for a longer period of time, perhaps to read or do some form of work in the evening. However, this artificial light was too dim to reset their biological clocks.[14] After the advent of electricity, artificial light played havoc with our natural rhythms.

Thomas Edison believed that people actually slept too much and that too much sleep was detrimental to their health. He envisioned that with the invention of the electric light bulb, people could extend their working hours and be more productive.[15] Sleep research conducted since the middle of the twentieth century has shown that Edison was wrong in that regard. Sleep deprivation does not lead to better productivity. To the contrary, we need to be rested and alert to be most productive. Margaret Thatcher and Thomas Edison were known to be insomniacs. But this was inaccurate. They functioned well with less than the average amount of sleep at night. Edison was known to take several naps during the day.[16]

There are definitely variations in the amount of sleep needed among individuals. Most of us probably know some people that get along well on six, five, or even fewer hours of sleep each night and who function well during the day. Other people who get this amount of sleep or less do not function well and do not feel good the next day—such as in my case. Why are there such variations? This is not really understood, but there is a great deal of information in the following chapters. It will be helpful to first understand what normal sleep is all about.

CHAPTER 2

Normal Sleep

By day's end, when the sun goes down, most of us are ready for a good night's sleep—hopefully, this will happen. You may ask, "What constitutes a good night's sleep?" The amount of sleep we strive for may be different from what we actually get. Also, the amount of sleep needed and achieved differs among individuals, as does the timing of people's sleep-wake cycles. Many of us proclaim, "I am a night person" or "I am a morning person." Some people are both—they like to go to bed late and get up early. I (Phyllis) used to be a "morning" person; and now (somewhat retired), I still go to bed fairly early (about 9:30 or 10:00 at night) and generally wake up between 6:30 and 7:00. About once a week, my husband and I go out to dinner, or a piano lounge, or dancing, often staying out past my usual bedtime. I still wake up about the same time in the morning.

So, what is this mysterious thing called sleep and what comprises a normal night's sleep? According to Dr. William Dement, a pioneer in the study of sleep science, "sleep erects a perceptual wall between the conscious mind and the outside world, and ... it is immediately reversible."[1] When a person is sleeping, he or she can be aroused—although this might be difficult if the individual is in deep sleep. This is the distinguishing feature between the sleep state and the unconscious state. Being in a coma or under anesthesia are examples of an unconscious state. Sleep is a natural state, while coma and anesthesia are unnatural states.

Why is sleep necessary? We know we don't function very well or even can't live without it, but scientists don't know exactly why this is so. Scientific investigations have shown that there are consequences to prolonged sleep deprivation. Important processes happen in our brains and body while we sleep. For example, growth hormone is secreted by our pituitary gland (located at the base of our brain) while we sleep. This hormone is responsible for body growth and repair of damaged body tissues. It is secreted in greater amounts in children who are still growing, and in lesser amounts in adults. In adults it is still needed for tissue repair.

It is still a mystery as to why sleep is so important. According to D. T. Max, "We know we miss it if we don't have it. And we know that no matter how much we try to resist it, sleep conquers us in the end."[2] For the most part, if we get about seven or eight hours of sleep each night, we wake up refreshed and are ready to do whatever we need to do. Then, about 15 to 17 hours later, we are ready to go to sleep again. There has been much speculation and research in the attempt to discern the importance of sleep. "Such studies suggest that memory consolidation may be one function of sleep.... So the purpose of sleep may be to help us remember what's important, by letting us forget what's not."[3] We've also established that growth and tissue restoration occur while we sleep. Sleep patterns vary from person to person. Some people get along fine on much less sleep than the average per night (or day) and seem to function very well.

According to Dr. Meir H. Kryger, past president of the American Academy of Sleep Medicine, although we really don't know why we sleep, we do know we feel rotten the next day and function poorly if we don't sleep. All animals need sleep. Laboratory animals that are deprived of sleep for long periods of time die.[4]

There currently is no specific scientific explanation of why adequate sleep is so important. There are theories, however. Explanations have focused on concepts of body restoration, energy conservation, and memory consolidation. There is also increasing evidence that sleep regulates body hormones, immunological functions, the cardiovascular system, and other body systems. It is known that the circadian system, in addition to regulating sleep and wake cycles, also regulates body temperature, hormonal systems, and other body processes.[5]

Why do humans sleep mostly at night instead of during daytime hours? Why do some animals sleep during the day and stay awake during the night? We do know that nocturnal animals hunt and survive better at night. Their genetic constitution allows them to better survive in their own habitats. Therefore, their biological clocks are different than the human clock for reasons of survival. On the other hand, our human forebears survived better by sleeping at night in a safe place and hunting and doing their work during daylight hours.

All animals (including the human animal), have inherent biological clocks that are synchronized to the 24 hours in which the earth rotates. (However, the human clock is slightly longer than 24 hours.) It is the solar light and darkness that determines our sleep patterns, or more specifically, sets our biological clocks. When we talk about our biological clocks, we are referring to neurological and hormonal processes in our brains and bodies that regulate our sleep-wake states and other body processes.

Biological clocks and circadian rhythms work together, but are two different processes. The "clock" refers to the regulating mechanisms (cells and chemicals in our brains and bodies) that control our sleep-wake cycle and other body processes, such as body temperature. The so-called "master clock" is located in the hypothalamus, a structure that lies at the base of the brain, just above the crossing of the optic nerves. It coordinates all our body clocks so they are in synch. This "master clock" is actually a "pea-sized" piece of brain tissue, consisting of about 20,000 nerve cells, referred to as the suprachiasmatic nuclei (SCN).[6] The SCN is the "awake" center (mentioned in Chapter 1), which responds to light. When daylight enters our eyes, it sends a "wake-up call" (by way of chemical and nerve transmission) to the SCN. The sleep center is a "pin-sized" cluster of cells, referred to as the ventrolateral preoptic nucleus (VLPO), which is also located in a structure at the base of the brain, close to the SCN. The VLPO sends signals to the SCN to stop producing its chemicals that keep us awake, when it is time for us to sleep. At the same time, another nearby structure, the pineal gland, secretes the hormone melatonin, which responds to darkness. Melatonin produces a calming effect, inducing sleep. Other brain structures also play a role during the various stages of sleep.[7]

In sum, the biological clock in the brain consists of a wake center and a sleep-inducing center. Our biological clock drives our circadian rhythms, which sets our sleep-wake cycle. The circadian rhythm tells our brain when to sleep and when to awaken. It is influenced by the earth's rotation of sunlight and darkness, which dictates the timing of when we sleep and when we wake up. Light is the main cue that sets our circadian rhythm. Genes also direct our biological clock functions and circadian rhythms.[8]

Our biological clock is actually longer than 24 hours. An early experiment conducted in 1938 provided evidence that this is so. A group of volunteers (all men) resided in a mammoth cave in Kentucky. This cave was a huge subterranean labyrinth of rooms and passageways with a constant temperature of 54 degrees Fahrenheit and was in total darkness. The volunteers ate when they were hungry, slept when they were sleepy, and woke naturally. There were no environmental cues, such as light or clocks. What happened was that the men went to bed an hour later than the previous night each night and woke an hour later each day. By the end of the week they were going to bed seven hours later than people "above them in the external world." What was learned was that, if unhindered by external cues, such as sunlight, the sleep-wake cycle is repeated every 25 to 26 hours, instead of 24 hours.[9]

There is also a homeostatic process that regulates the amount and timing of when we sleep and when we wake up. The homeostatic process is an internal pressure that begins from the time we awake in the morning and increases throughout the day. "People cannot remain awake effectively for extended periods, nor can they sleep indefinitely." This homeostatic pressure becomes more marked in people who are sleep deprived.[10]

To sum up, our sleep-wake cycle (circadian rhythm) is regulated internally by our biological clock and is externally influenced by the light and dark cycle of the earth's rotation. When light enters the eyes, the retina sends an "alerting" message to the SCN in the hypothalamus. Magically, we wake up. This is the circadian process.

As stated earlier, the neurological and hormonal processes that regulate our circadian rhythm also regulate other body functions, such as our internal body temperature and metabolism. These processes fluctuate in rhythms synchronized with our sleep-awake cycles. This is how the process starts. Sunlight stimulates nerve transmission from the retina (in back of our eyes) to the suprachiasmatic nucleus (SCN) in the hypothalamus. From this structure, the message is sent (via nerve pathways) to our pituitary gland. The pituitary gland then secretes adrenocortico-trophic hormone (ACTH) (one of several hormones secreted by this "master" gland). ACTH travels to our adrenal glands (located above each kidney), which, in turn, secrete cortisol and other hormones responsible for several metabolic processes in our bodies.[11]

One of the functions of cortisol is to keep us alert, so that we can be productive during the day. We are then aroused and remain alert and productive when our world is lit up by natural light (assuming we have slept well the night before). Greater amounts of cortisol, along with adrenalin (also secreted by our adrenal glands), are produced when we are stressed or encounter danger to prepare our bodies for "fight or flight." For example, when I (Phyllis) can't fall asleep, I worry about not sleeping (the danger). My pituitary gland sends out ACTH to my adrenal glands, which then secrete adrenalin and cortisol. I am then aroused when I am supposed to feel calm and sleepy; a vicious cycle ensues. This is probably one explanation for other people who have difficulty falling asleep. Cortisol and adrenalin have the opposite effect of another hormone that plays a role in calming us down and preparing us for sleep—melatonin.

The pineal gland, located near the hypothalamus and pituitary gland, synthesizes and secretes melatonin. The secretion of this hormone, which helps us fall asleep, is controlled by the circadian clock and occurs in darkness. Melatonin ceases to be synthesized when sufficient light enters the room.[12] This mechanism explains why many people who work night shifts or travel across time zones have difficulty sleeping until their biological clocks readjust—which takes time.

Shift work is a recent invention—since the Industrial Revolution. The huge factories in that era took a long time to heat up, so they had to keep the furnaces going all day and night, setting the stage for night-shift work. However, since our clocks are set for night sleeping and daytime alertness, this became a problem. Since humans cannot sleep at will, night workers quickly build up significant sleep debt. The body eventually adapts, but it takes time. It is particularly problematic for people working swing shifts— working nights for a short period, then switching to day or evening shifts, and back again to night shifts.[13]

Although shift work increases productivity and customer service, it has inherent health and safety risks. Of course it is of absolute necessity in such work places as hospitals and police forces. Shift workers build up large amounts of sleep debt, which can lead to significant health problems and present high risks of injury to self and others. According to the National Sleep Foundation, "If you are a shift worker and have difficulty sleeping during the day, chances are you also have difficulty staying awake at work. Also, the more sleepy you are, the more likely you are to experience a 'microsleep,' an involuntary bout of sleep brought on by sleep deprivation that lasts for a few seconds."[14] As a nurse, I am very much aware of this issue. I only worked night duty two nights a week for one year, in 1968, when my youngest child was in first grade. We only had one car, so the plan was that I worked at night and got home in the morning in time for my husband to take the car to work. Since I slept the night before my first scheduled night shift, I couldn't sleep during the day. I tried to take a nap, but was unable to fall asleep. So I went to work, not having slept since the night before. By morning I had to struggle to stay awake and alert. I was, after all, responsible for sick people. When I got home, I had to help get the kids off to school and finally got to bed about nine or ten in the morning. Guess what? I couldn't get to sleep for hours. To make matters worse, we had a dog which I kept in our fenced yard. Linus thought he was a cat and climbed the fence. On one occasion, after about two hours of sleep, a nice neighbor called me to tell me my dog was roaming about. Then, I had to go back to work that second night. I did not fare well that year. When the year ended, my children said to me, "Mommy, you're not going to work nights anymore, are you?" I think you get the picture. We bought a second car.

Because the sun has such a powerful influence on our sleep-wake cycle, it is difficult to sleep during the day. To make matters worse, well-meaning friends, relatives, neighbors, and other people (telemarketers) tend to call during the day, when they are awake. As a result, shift workers suffer from sleep deprivation—they are irritable, moody, and very tired. Some tips are to try to avoid swing shifts, make your bedroom as dark as possible, go to sleep a little later each night for several days before your night shift begins, and remind as many people as possible not to disturb you on days you need to sleep.[15]

Another disruption of our sleep-wake cycle can be traveling through different time zones. Our internal clock conflicts with the new time zone. People who travel are quite familiar with the signs of jet lag. If we travel eastward—for example, from the United States to Europe—we generally travel at night and arrive at our destination in the morning. By our clocks, it is evening—time for bed. Those people who are fortunate enough to sleep on the plane have an easier time adjusting. I am not one who can do this, as I revealed my own plight with jet lag in Chapter 1.

According to Dr. J. Paul Caldwell, in his book, *Sleep*, it is easier to travel westward because westward flights lengthen the day—effectively, one is in daylight longer before bedtime—and our circadian sleep-wake cycle tends to be slightly longer than 24 hours, as I mentioned earlier.[16] For some unknown reason, I also had a difficult time traveling home, westward-bound from Israel. Caldwell suggests the following tips to decrease the effects of jet lag[17]:

• Gradually shift your sleeping and eating schedules toward your destination arrival time.
• Drink lots of fluids, but avoid caffeinated beverages and alcohol.
• Switch your watch and clock to the new arrival time of your destination.
• If all else fails, take a short-acting hypnotic for a short period of time—which is what I did. Also, try taking melatonin to help you fall asleep.

Another characteristic of our normal circadian rhythm is that there are peaks and troughs during the 24-hour cycle. Once we wake up in the morning, we do not necessarily keep going strong all day long. There is a cycle of rising and falling levels of alertness throughout the day, due to some fluctuations of hormonal secretions, which vary during the day. As a result, we feel sleepy during certain times of the day. Usually, our periods of greatest alertness occur mid-morning, between nine and eleven. In general, the lowest period of alertness occurs between three and five o'clock in the morning, with a second trough occurring mid-afternoon.[18] This explains why all through my early nursing school days and later college and graduate school days, I had such a difficult time staying awake in classes following lunch. In some countries, such as in Spain and Latin America, people take afternoon siestas. Then people are more alert and productive when they return to work.

Another burning question is how much sleep do we need when we retire for the night (or day)? It is known that some people seem to get along with five hours or less without feeling sleep-deprived the next day. Others don't feel rested and refreshed unless they get at least seven or eight hours of sleep.

In a study conducted in 1993 at the National Institutes of Health, healthy subjects were kept in a dark room from dusk to dawn. The subjects had no underlying sleep disorders, nor were they taking any medications or substances. The results were that they slept on an average of eight hours and fifteen minutes.[19]

What happens when we go to sleep? As mentioned earlier, sleep is a relatively young science. In times past, it was a mysterious state and still is to a large extent. Philosophers speculated that people actually died during sleep and returned to life when they awakened. Freud theorized about dreams. In his book, *The Interpretation of Dreams*, "Freud proposed that dreams disguise forbidden thoughts or desires by cloaking them in other forms."[20] It is presently believed that dreams do not reveal our true thoughts and emotions. Dr. Dement states, "The brain takes what is essentially random, meaningless nerve activation and 'synthesizes' something that has some meaning and coherence even if it has to resort to making up its own story. Accordingly, there is no hidden meaning in dreams."[21] Based on later-twentieth-century scientific data, Freud was wrong. In his later years, Freud acknowledged that he was not sure about his theories. However, he was a pioneer in stimulating research into human psychology.

The mysteries of sleep and their disorders have been somewhat revealed from knowledge gained by scientific studies since the mid–twentieth century. Early studies involved the placement of electrodes on areas of people's heads in controlled laboratory environments. These electrodes were hooked up to a machine to record electrical impulses of the human brain. These recordings are now well-known as electroencephalograms (EEG). Sleep studies are still conducted using EEG tracings to identify stages of sleep, which are described a few pages below. Other sleep tests performed in a sleep lab include electromyogram (EMG), electrooculogram (EOG), electrocardiogram (ECG), respiratory monitoring, audiovisual monitoring, and multiple sleep latency test (MSLT). Collectively, these laboratory tests are referred to as polysomnograms.

The EMG test records electrical activity in skeletal muscles to detect the occurrence of muscle twitching. The EOG measures eye movements to detect when in the sleep cycle rapid eye movements (REM) occurs. The ECG records the heart's electrical activity. Audiovisual monitoring allows the practitioner to monitor sleep behaviors and sounds in "time-synchronized" manner in order to evaluate abnormalities in a particular stage of sleep. The MSLT is a daytime test involving 4 to 5 brief nap opportunities that measures an average of how long it takes a person to fall asleep.[22]

The subjects of such sleep studies have generally been volunteers, such as medical students or even those scientists conducting the research. EEG recordings reveal various wave forms that occur during sleep for a period of time. These wave forms are repeated in cycles several times during an approximately eight-hour period of sleep. It was discovered that these wave forms were different from EEG recordings on subjects who were awake. During wakefulness, the wave forms show high frequencies, but low voltage and amplitude, and are referred to as beta waves. Each of the wave forms that occur during sleep are noted as a given stage of sleep. There are five stages that occur in a given sleep cycle. Four of these stages are non–REM sleep and the fifth stage is noted as REM sleep. If you observe someone sleeping, you can actually see the subject's eyes moving under his or her lids. This is the stage of sleep when dreams occur.

There is a "pre-stage of sleep, characterized by wave forms that are lower in frequency and of higher amplitude than the beta waves. Dr. Dement describes this stage as a very calm state when the person is totally relaxed, just prior to the onset of true sleep. The wave forms of this stage are called alpha waves.[23]

I have always told my husband that I can never really fall asleep during the day or while in the car (as passenger). However, I do believe I occasionally go into the alpha state. I'm aware of what is going on in my environment, but am in such a state of calmness, I am unable to respond to conversation or other mild stimuli. And, in spite of my protestations, I probably do cross over to the first stage of sleep on rare occasions.

When the alpha waves change to the even slower frequency and higher-amplitude wave forms, called theta waves, the person has entered the first stage of sleep, which generally lasts about five to ten minutes. This stage is characterized by complete relaxation, although the person can be easily aroused. Stage two is moderately light sleep, in which there is a greater degree of muscle relaxation, slowing of heart rate and drop in body temperature. While in stage two, recorded brain waves are slower in frequency and are mixed with sporadic bursts of faster waves, called spindles (resembling spindles on an old spinning wheel), and K-complexes, which are large electrical discharges in the brain. In another five to ten minutes of stage two, the sleeper enters the third stage.[24]

The third stage of sleep is deep sleep. The brain emits wave forms that are of low frequency and high in amplitude, called delta waves. These wave forms are more regular than the theta waves. When these delta waves constitute most of the sleep during a measured sleep period, the sleeper is in the deepest sleep—that of stage four.

Stage four is characterized by muscle relaxation, decreased heart rate, slower and regular respiratory rate, and lower body temperature. It is difficult to arouse the person in this deepest of sleep stages. It is in this stage that growth-hormone is released from the pituitary gland and is responsible for growth in children and tissue repair in all ages. Some experts group stages three and four together. These stages may last for about 45 minutes and then, the sleeper usually shifts into REM sleep.[25]

As stated above, REM sleep is the stage in which dreaming occurs. The brain waves, as seen on the EEG tracing, resemble those of wakefulness. These waves are low in amplitude, but return to a fast frequency wave form, indicating that the brain is active and using a lot of energy. Imaging of the brain during a REM sleep stage shows an increase in blood flow to the brain. If the sleeper is observed carefully, the observer can see bursts of eye flutters and back and forth movements under the sleeper's eye lids.

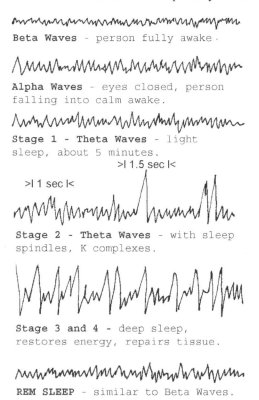

Beta Waves - person fully awake.

Alpha Waves - eyes closed, person falling into calm awake.

Stage 1 - Theta Waves - light sleep, about 5 minutes.

>| 1.5 sec |<

>| 1 sec |<

Stage 2 - Theta Waves - with sleep spindles, K complexes.

Stage 3 and 4 - deep sleep, restores energy, repairs tissue.

REM SLEEP - similar to Beta Waves.

Exhibit 1—Graphs of normal EEG signals when fully awake, and those entering and in sleep stages. The stages are described in the text. The graphs have been constructed from information in a number of the references, as cited. Briefly, the awake stage changes to an alpha stage, in which a calm, restful condition, perhaps with closed eyes, is achieved. An active EEG pattern is still observed. Often when not further disturbed, the person will pass into what most authors call Stage 1 of sleep, when theta waves will appear on an EEG, as indicated in the graphs. In Stage l, the person is no longer aware of his surroundings and can be said to be isolated from the outside world. However, he can still be easily awakened by even a whisper. He remains in Stage 1 for about five minutes before transitioning into Stage 2, which is a deeper sleep. Stage 2 can be distinguished in a sleep laboratory by a wave pattern that is often interrupted by a burst of more frequent waves called sleep spindles, followed after some further seconds by a sharp dip and sharper peak called K complexes, as shown in the graphs. The spindles and K complexes will repeat themselves while the patient remains in Stage 2, which is often only another five minutes or so. When the pattern changes to less frequent but much higher voltage waves (called "delta waves"), as shown in the graphs, then the patient is known to have entered "deep sleep," which is Stages 3 and 4, with similar wave patterns. Some experts just lump Stages 3 and 4 together in describing sleep patterns. In the above graphs, Stage 3 lasts for up to about 15 minutes and then transitions to Stage 4, with a very similar wave pattern. Stage 4 lasts for about 45 minutes in good sleep, and then changes to rapid eye movement (REM) sleep, with a wave pattern changing back almost to the same as the awake pattern. However, Stage 4 might sometimes return to Stage 3 for another 10 minutes or so, before REM stage is entered. This pattern will repeat itself four or five times, each for a cycle of 90 minutes or so, in normal sleep. However, sometimes REM sleep will return to deep sleep stages directly, or to Stages 1 or 2. Sometimes an alpha stage will be followed by REM sleep. The fraction of REM sleep decreases with age. As discussed in the text, deep sleep is when the energy is restored and tissue growth (in the young) or repair (healing) takes place. In REM sleep, the individual has dreams that often can be remembered when awakened naturally or by some disturbance; during the REM sleep, the individual is also paralyzed by nature against limb movement, presumably as designed to protect others from violent movements that might be induced by violent, terrorizing dreams. The books cited in references will discuss the many variations in this normal pattern. The variations can allow the physician or other sleep professional to diagnose, together with the other polysomnogram and medical indicators, the nature of a person's sleep problems and the possible remedies.

These movements were first observed at the University of Chicago's sleep lab in 1953, by Dr. Nathaniel Kleitman and his student, Eugene Aserinsky. These researchers observed these eye movements occurring at the same time that the EEG recording of wave forms changed from the slow wave (of deep delta sleep) to the characteristic wave form we now identify with REM sleep. Cells that lie in certain parts of our midbrain, called the pons, are stimulated during REM sleep. The nerve impulses then travel through the brain to the part that controls eye movements.[26] The pons also blocks signals to the spinal cord, which causes temporary paralysis of our skeletal (voluntary) muscles. This means that during REM sleep, people are unable to move their arms and legs. Apparently, this prevents us from acting out our dreams. Some people, however, do have an abnormal ability to move during REM, supposedly acting out their dreams. These unusual sleep patterns are referred to as parasomnias, which are discussed later in this book.

The association between REM sleep and dreams was first discovered in

1952, when Dr. Dement, as a second-year medical student working in Dr. Nathaniel Kleitman's sleep lab, monitored the EEG tracings on volunteer medical students. When the tracings signified changes in the pattern to that of REM sleep, he awakened the students and asked them if they were dreaming. Indeed, they were able to describe their dreams vividly.[27]

Science still doesn't understand all the mysteries of REM sleep and of dreams. It is unknown why, as active as the brain is during this stage, the muscles of the body (except for the autonomic muscles that control body functions such as breathing, blood pressure, etc.) are temporarily paralyzed. Another interesting occurrence during REM sleep is that men have been observed to have erections. Also, women have pelvic engorgement. (How this was measured is not described.) These occurrences are not believed to be related to erotic dreams, because penile erections can also be observed in infant boys.[28] Erections are not caused by muscle contractions; they are caused by blood engorgement.

REM sleep occurs more frequently and lasts longer in young children. It occupies about 50 percent of sleep time in the newborn and reduces to about 20 to 25 percent by about two years of age and continues at this rate into adulthood.[29] The first REM sleep usually lasts about ten minutes, then the dreamer drifts back into deep sleep. There are about four to six cycles of REM alternating with non–REM sleep stages throughout the night.[30]

A normal (or typical) sleep cycle does not proceed from stage 1 to REM and back again, which would seem logical. As sleep studies have shown, Stage 1 lasts up to 10 minutes, progressing to Stage 2, which can last 10 to 25 minutes. Stage 3 lasts from one to five minutes, quickly progressing to Stage 4, which lasts about 20 to 40 minutes. Then the sleeper returns to Stage 3 for a minute or two, back to Stage 2 for another five to ten minutes, and then to the first REM sleep. REM sleep begins about 60 to 90 minutes from the onset of sleep. These cycles are repeated about every 90 minutes throughout the night. Stages 3 and 4 are longest during the early cycles, get shorter as the night progresses, and may drop out altogether in later cycles. Stage 2 and REM sleep last longer in later cycles.[31]

This so-called "normal" or "typical" sleep pattern changes with age and is influenced by environmental disturbances, medical problems, travel, stress, and a myriad of sleep disorders. Also, sleep disturbances are common in women prior to and during menstruation, in pregnancy, menopause, and post-menopause. The following chapters will explore the many underlying causes of insomnia and unusual sleep disturbances.

Chapter 3

The Authors' Stories

In this chapter, the authors, Phyllis and Allen, will tell their own personal stories and experiences with sleep. They will each tell their own histories of sleep patterns throughout their respective lives, as well as their observations and perceptions of the sleep patterns of each other. In this way, some of the many changes in each author's sleep patterns can be related, in the years after their wedding, to the other's perceptions of, and problems with, the mate's sleep problems. Because of the long years of life of both authors and the many changes in their life situations, it is possible that many readers will relate their own experiences to many of those of the authors. These stories may also be used as examples of sleep problems described in other chapters of the book. Perhaps more entertaining, the reader might also find, in the authors' stories, some humorous material that provides insights related to the reader's own personal experiences. Enjoy, and be part of our family.

Phyllis's Experience (as Told by Phyllis)

Sleep has been an issue with me as far back as I can remember. I did not experience insomnia as a child. I do remember that my environment had to be just so—quiet, dark, calm—for me to fall asleep. My sister often kept her radio on too loud, preventing my ability to be calm (yes, before we had a TV, although it was on the market). If she so obliged, I then was able to fall asleep. I had recurring nightmares (which I remember to this day). There was a dog sitting in one corner of my room, looking at me with wide eyes. He would then get up and start to move toward me, at which point I woke up screaming. My mother would comfort me and then I fell back to sleep. I think this only occurred once during the night and not every night. I don't remember how long a time that these dreams lasted. The strange part of it was that I was never afraid of dogs. We never had one because my sister had a terrible phobia of dogs and cats.

I had one episode of sleepwalking as a preteen that I can remember. I don't remember if there were others, but the memory of this event remained with me all of these years. I was babysitting for my next door neighbors' two children. We lived on a street of row houses and all the neighbors on our street knew each other, as if we were a very large extended family. I believe I was only about eleven years old, but capable and knew the children since their birth. They were preschool age at the time.

The children were fast asleep upstairs, while I was watching television in the living room. I fell asleep on their sofa. I was in my pajamas because I was sleeping over. The next thing I knew was I was outside their front door. I do remember saying to myself that "I had to go home." I tried to get back in, but I had locked myself out. At that point, I was fully awake and began to panic. I went next door to my home, but my parents and sister were not at home and the door was locked. I then ran to the neighbors' house on the other side and they were home. Embarrassed by my being in my pajamas and by what had happened, I just explained the situation. The husband was able to climb into a basement window and then open the door for me. I was so grateful and relieved. Of course I told my neighbors and parents what happened. I don't remember their reaction and don't remember them being overly concerned. I don't recall another incident of that nature recurring.

I do not remember having any difficulty sleeping for the remainder of my teen years until I entered nursing school in 1954. During the second half of that first year, we started going onto the hospital units to "practice" our nursing skills on "real" people. During these clinical rotations, we had to be on our assigned units at 7 A.M. sharp. It was not easy falling asleep at night during these times, although we did have our own rooms in the dormitory. We were on duty for four hours, then we went to lunch, and then we attended classroom lectures for four hours in the afternoon. This was the clincher— how to stay awake during these lectures? I mainly fell asleep during Mrs. O'Brian's lectures on pharmacology.

After being caught several times with my eyes closed and head wobbling, I was called to her office. She asked me if I was getting enough sleep. I explained to her that I definitely tried to. She said, "Perhaps if you were grounded on weekends, you might catch up." I told her I would try harder, which I did, but it was a struggle.

Later, in the three-year nursing program, I did have to do some evening and night shifts. Fortunately this was not too frequently, because I had an extremely difficult time sleeping during the day. It was especially difficult during a two-month rotation to a communicable disease hospital in Philadelphia. I was on night duty for about two weeks. Our dorm rooms were actually cubicles—open walls at the top. I heard the women filling the ice bins and any other sound clearly. I don't know how I survived those weeks. But, somehow I did.

After I was graduated from nursing school in 1957, I was fortunate enough to work day or evening shifts. I married my high school boyfriend while still in training, during my senior year of nurse training. We lived in my parents' home. There were times during my early married years (to my first husband) that I began to have difficulty falling asleep. He was also going to school and he either studied in bed or watched television (which was in our bedroom). It was difficult for me to fall asleep with the lights and television on.

I always seemed to need a lot of sleep (how many hours I didn't think about) and frequently felt quite tired the next day. After each of my three children were born, as most new parents have to contend with, it was difficult getting up at night to feed my babies. Fortunately, all three began to sleep through the night at three months of age.

As time went on, I had more and more difficulty falling asleep at night. It didn't help that my first husband and I had many arguments and he continued to have the TV on until after the 11 P.M. news. I would doze, but be wide awake when he finally turned off the TV. I was exhausted and wanted only to fall asleep. There was a lot of stress in that marriage.

Throughout those years I had difficulty falling asleep. There were also nights that I lay awake the entire night. It so happened that my first husband was a pharmacist, who, in the ensuing years after our marriage, earned master's and doctor's degrees in neuropharmacology. He didn't think I should take sleeping pills. I just struggled through those years and took afternoon naps if I had the time. When my children were preteens, I returned to school to obtain my B.S. in nursing, then my M.S.—more stress! I graduated in 1979 and then taught nursing in various colleges and universities for the next 20 years.

My first marriage ended in 1981. The break-up was initiated by my husband. The first few nights after my husband announced his intentions, I didn't sleep at all. It was particularly difficult because I was teaching and had to be alert for my teaching responsibilities. If I was able to finally fall asleep, I would wake as early as 3 or 4 in the morning, which lasted for several months.

During my period of grieving, I still remember some strange dreams I had. Dreams are mysterious and still puzzle many an expert. Although some experts believe that dreams do not reveal true thoughts or hidden meaning, I believe they may be symbolic of our emotions. After my first husband left, I was going for counseling. I related to her about a dream I had. My former husband and I were making love and I told him to "take off your toupee." This was strange to me, because it never bothered him that he was somewhat bald and never even thought about a toupee. She asked me if I thought I was asking him to "remove his façade." This was a "wow" moment, because I never really did know who he was in all of our 25 years of marriage.

Another dream I still remember was that, in my dream, my husband and I were going shopping with my youngest (17-year-old) daughter and getting out of the car. All of the sudden, Lisa was gone. I woke up petrified. Down deep, I think I was afraid of also losing her.

I remarried in 1984. Allen and I were happy together, but there were other stressors in our lives. Allen had a very ill son. My mother was ill and died shortly after we were married. I had a very stressful job as manager of a hospital department. My insomnia had worsened. I did finally seek help and talked to my gynecologist, who prescribed Valium if I was unable to sleep. Valium is not an ideal drug for sleeping. For one thing, it is addicting. It can cause dizziness, tremors, confusion, depression, hallucinations, and other adverse effects. The Valium helped me sleep, but I still felt groggy the next day. I tried other things, such as relaxation exercises. I actually taught these techniques to couples in my Childbirth Preparation classes. They just didn't work for me. What a hypocrite I was.

I resigned from the managerial position and accepted a new position at Providence Hospital as a clinical educator. I enjoyed this position, which I held for five years; then things changed. I accepted a new (similar) position at another hospital, but after the first two weeks, realized I made a terrible mistake by resigning from Providence Hospital. I know what you're think-ing—we all have stress in our lives. This, of course, is true; insomnia is usu-ally exacerbated at times of increased stress in our lives.

Allen and I had planned to move to Ocean Pines, which we had visited while vacationing in Ocean City, Maryland. We had already decided we would do this when we retired. I was way too young to retire, but there were advantages to the move. We were able to sell our house in Rockville and buy one in Ocean Pines. Allen had already retired from the government and was doing consulting and part time teaching at Georgetown University. I could find another position. We moved in December 1990. We started packing and getting rid of excess possessions.

In the meantime, my insomnia was getting worse. My doctor was con-cerned about continuing my prescription for Valium and suggested I see a psychiatrist. I agreed, anything to help. I was feeling depressed—because of lack of sleep, or the Valium, or a combination of both. Either way, I needed help. Three days prior to the move I couldn't sleep at all.

The psychiatrist was a very caring woman. Just talking to her made me feel better. She put me on the lowest dosage of doxepin (Sinequan), which is an anti-depressant and is also therapeutic for sleep disorders. I've been taking this medicine nightly and will continue to do so. It has helped regulate my sleep. However, there are still times I am unable to fall asleep or can't fall back to sleep if I awake during the night.

After we were settled into our new home, I was writing nursing standards for a fellow nurse entrepreneur. I was commissioned to present all-day workshops on these standards in two middle states—back-to-back. I flew in the day before, checked into the hotel, ate dinner, and checked to see if my supplies had arrived. By the time I got to bed, I couldn't sleep the entire night. I took three doxepins. They didn't work. I did not function very well the next day and the participant evaluations of my presentation were terrible. At the end of the workshop, I traveled to the next state. I slept better that night and my presentation was better. I still felt lousy.

When I related this scenario to my psychiatrist, she ordered a backup sleeping medication, which I try not to take too often. Just knowing that I have this backup helps me to stay calmer and sleep better. However, it is there if I need it. After we settled into our new home, there were still many nights when I was unable to fall asleep. Our new primary care physician continued to prescribe doxepin, and Zolpidem (Ambien) as a backup. I try not to take the Ambien too often. I especially need it when I travel or visit family.

If I don't get the amount of sleep my body seems to need, I feel tired, sleepy, and irritable the next day. I am unable to fall asleep during the day if I try to take a nap. My daily schedule is usually full, either exercising, writing, attending organization meetings, subbing as a school nurse, giving a course, or doing yard work in the spring and fall. Even if I lose sleep, I still push myself to do what I had planned for that day. Some days it is difficult, but regardless of sleep deficit, I am self-driven to do what I had planned to do.

Allen's Experience (as Told by Phyllis)

Allen does not believe he has insomnia. However, I've been sleeping with him for a long time (married at this writing for almost 26 years). He may not have insomnia, but he certainly has some strange sleeping habits. His body clock is different from mine. I prefer getting into bed by 8:30 or

9:00 P.M. and reading for awhile. Once in a while, Allen does the same. But then, after about two or three hours of sleep, he often wakes up and is unable to go back to sleep. So he will get up and read, watch television, or write (whatever he is working on at the time). The reason he doesn't think he has insomnia is because he doesn't let it bother him as it does me if I'm unable to get a good night's sleep. Unlike me, he is able to sleep later in the morning (sometimes past noon) or take naps during the day.

Allen works better in the afternoon, evening, or during the night. Whatever I'm working on, my brain shuts off about 5 P.M., whereas Allen's starts functioning. Of course, he is somewhat retired and so can be flexible in his routine. For an old man, his mind and body are still active. In the early years of our marriage (he was then middle-aged), for the most part, he slept through the night and still took "cat naps" during the day, at times—even at work. He would shut his office door and prop his feet up on the desk.

Throughout our marriage, Allen snored. This only exacerbated my insomnia. At times I got used to it, used ear plugs, or told him to turn the other way. It is interesting that often he obeyed me without waking up, or if he did, he went right back to sleep. There were times when I was awake and thought he had some sleep apnea. Watching him carefully, I noted he stopped breathing for seconds (I didn't count) and then gasp. When I confronted him with this observation, he denied this. But, after a time, he lost some weight and that problem seemed to have corrected itself.

For the past several years, he hasn't snored as frequently and if he does, it's much softer. If he is facing me, his heavy breathing can keep me awake, which I have told him. Of course, he comes back with, "Do you want me to stop breathing?" "No," I respond; "I just want you to turn over."

Whatever amount of sleep Allen is able to get, he gets up to play tennis in good weather. Then he will nap during the day. If it is raining or too cold, he skips tennis and sleeps until he feels ready to get up. Being retired, he feels he can sleep when he chooses and work (basically writing) when he pleases. He doesn't believe in sleeping pills and would never resort to taking them. Because of his lifestyle, it is hard to say whether or not he has insomnia. He does compensate for the most part, but I do believe he accumulates significant sleep debt at times.

Phyllis's Experience (as Told by Allen)

Having known Phyllis since I fell in love with her after meeting her at a dance party on December 11, 1981, and then marrying her on March 16, 1984

(I better remember that date), I have seen and intimately experienced some changes in her patterns and attitudes about her sleep. Of course, I cannot describe Phyllis' sleep patterns before the time I met her. The reader has available her own descriptions of sleep experiences before I met her, when she was in her mid-forties and I had recently turned 53.

In writing this, it occurs to me that changes in our sleep patterns have been affected by changes in life situations and experiences. (This is consistent with Neubauer's fourth perspective to employ in diagnosing sleep disorders: the lifestyle aspects of the patient.) I will go into more of the types of life experiences that have affected my sleep habits in the next section describing my recollections of how sleep changed during my life cycle. However, there is not room here for entire personal autobiographies. It will suffice for the readers of this book if I begin by reviewing the changes in the emotional and romantic settings that Phyllis and I experienced since meeting at mid-life, with some additional embellishment with pertinent and related changes in family, job, professional, and recreational situations as we progressed toward our "retirement" years. These changes all affected our sleep patterns.

First, let us consider how Phyllis and I met. We met at an Open University dance at a Friday night dance party in a studio on Connecticut Avenue in Washington, D.C. After I had danced a few with my date of the evening, the dance instructor started a Paul Jones dance of changing partners. When the music stopped the second time for changing partners, I heard someone behind me say, "I'm going to grab somebody." I liked the sound of her voice, swiveled around, and said, "Grab me, grab me!" I immediately liked her looks, the way she talked, and the way she danced with me. I also learned she was a nurse and seemed caring and intelligent. I told her I was in the Montgomery County telephone directory and gave her my name; I asked her to call me, thinking she would not want to give her name and telephone number to a stranger. However, she told me her name and that her telephone number was in the directory under the name of her ex-husband, who had departed only six months before. I was impressed that she seemed relatively together for only a six-month separation and resolved to soon call her. I now know that this chance meeting with Phyllis initiated a profound change in my lifestyle and future sleep patterns.

After meeting Phyllis for that minute on a Friday evening, I went home with the date I had taken to the dance. However, I was then already thinking that I must look up the telephone number of Phyllis and call her soon. On Sunday morning, less than two days later, I was in the bathtub planning to call her as soon as I dressed. However, before I left the tub to call Phyllis, the telephone rang and my housemate told me that Phyllis was calling. I was wringing wet. I told him to hold the telephone, threw a towel around me, and left the bathroom to answer the call. I liked the sound of her voice, and I liked the way she talked. I also liked that she called me first, because it meant that perhaps I also had some appeal to her. When I talked with her, I soon asked for a date the next Friday night at the Shoreham Hotel in D.C., to listen to the humor of Mark Russell, dine, and dance to a big band. Things were really swinging in Washington, D.C., in those days of the early 1980s.

After hanging up the telephone, I realized that I wanted to get to know her sooner, so I called her back and arranged to meet her for pizza the following night. We met for pizza near her home, and talked for several hours. She was very attractive and personable to me. I found her so caring about her own family and compassionate about some of mine, as well as the patients she had cared for as a nurse. (Also, I think I realized subconsciously that as I was aging I might need the love of a good nurse.)

I was already falling in love as we entered the Shoreham Hotel the following Friday evening. After Mark Russell finished his humorous show in the Shoreham lounge, there was a wait of about a half-hour before the dining and music room opened. I noticed a beautiful, large, concert grand piano in the lobby waiting area about ninety feet away; it was surrounded with comfortable looking sofas. I cannot resist the sight of a beautiful grand piano. I beckoned to Phyllis to follow me to one of these sofas. I then sat at the piano singing Phyllis a few old love songs, hoping this would further uplift her attraction to me. Then, we went in to dine and dance, and found we moved and fit well together on the dance floor. The night ended beautifully with the beginning of our love affair.

The date at the Shoreham thus began to solidify the romantic aspects of my life and change my own sleep patterns. (I have written a song about that, dedicated to Phyllis.) I suspect that Phyllis also had become attracted to me at that time, and that this has at least somewhat affected her sleep patterns from then on, as I will describe here. When two people begin to live together, they each usually experience at least some changes in their lifestyles and sleep patterns.

What I observed during over two years of courtship was that Phyllis, normally an early-to-bed, early-to-rise morning person, did seem to enjoy staying up sometimes to the wee hours in the morning on weekend dates where we could listen to music and sing or dance. Of course, on weekends, she did not need to arise early for work. She told me that she had not had this kind of weekend fun previously. Thus, on these weekends she often became a night person, getting a "second wind" in the evenings. She seemed, even with some sleep loss, to still perform well in her teaching duties during the week at the University of Maryland School of Nursing.

As the years of our marriage went by, it seemed that, more and more,

Phyllis preferred to establish a more regular schedule of going to bed between 8:30 and 9:30 P.M., and reading until becoming sleepy, gradually refraining from other bedtime activities, television or otherwise, that would be stimulating and prevent her from falling asleep. The exception to this has been our regular Saturday night dates, New Year's Eve, and sometimes other special occasions, when she will enjoy an evening out, for dining, singing, dancing, and/or attending entertaining theater arts or concerts. I cannot complain about her sleep habits; she is a wonderful, loving wife, and is still beautiful to this old octogenarian. I am still in heaven in her arms, whenever I can get there.

As I see it, her sleep problems now include mainly: (1) she often wakes up after only a few hours sleep and then worries about her sleep so much that she needs to take a sleeping pill to sleep again; (2) she then worries the next morning that she needed to take a pill, and feels guilty; (3) she is more or less tired the next day after taking a pill; (4) she then worries about being tired, because she likes to be productive during the day, and at the same time keep up with all home chores and finish any projects or assignments (which she takes on as a giving and sharing person) well before any deadlines; (5) then she worries whether I will do all of the chores and projects that she expects me to before any crises of failure, as she sees it, might occur; and finally, (6) she again worries before going to sleep whether she will be able to sleep through the night without taking a pill. So, to me, much of her sleep problems, call it a form of insomnia, result from the fact that she worries too much about her sleep. After all, she is still here, in great shape, and relatively healthy for a semi-retired nurse in her seventies. Her worries about sleep are further amplified by the fact that she worries about everything else.

Although she used to complain that snoring kept her awake, and she would wake me and make me turn to the other side, she does not do so anymore. As indicated in the next section, a few years ago, I deliberately lost 22 pounds so I could move faster on the tennis courts. After that, she said that any snoring I did was not so loud, and that my sleep apnea had disappeared. I think that she has finally adapted to my sleep habits, and that I do not disturb her much, even when I sneak into or out of bed.

However, she often dreams and talks or mumbles in phrases I cannot understand, when she is in REM sleep. She also sometimes hollers loudly when dreaming so that I often am worried about her, and need to talk to her to wake her or calm her down. Once not too long ago she hollered, "Allen, stop snoring!" This time, I had been awake for a couple of hours, thinking about things with my eyes closed and occasionally hearing her (until then quiet) snore, content that she was sleeping. I said, "Phyllis, I have been awake for about two hours thinking and not snoring. It was *your* own *loud* snoring, just now, that woke you up!" Fortunately, she believed me; otherwise no argument would have helped.

I have tried to tell Phyllis not to worry about her sleep, so that it might ease her mind. However, I have found it is of no use to tell Phyllis not to worry; she just gets mad. I guess she feels I should know that worry about sleep is a natural part of her female physiology, psychology, and life altogether.

An important clarification regarding my feelings about Phyllis' sleep problems: Any noises, gentle snoring, or sleep talking that comes from Phyllis' side of the bed when I am awake is music to my ears! I am just so happy that she is sleeping, and will not feel so tired and grumpy the next day, that her noises do not bother me, and are not the cause of my remaining awake. If I am asleep when she makes her lovely noises, then I am not aware of them and they do not wake me up.

Well, you can read Phyllis' accounts of these matters; she is honest about her observations and feelings. Some reference back to these paragraphs about Phyllis, and with perhaps some further revelations, might later become informative.

Phyllis, please sleep in good health, any way you can. It will be a joy to us both!

Allen's Experience (as Told by Allen)

I will tell my experiences as I remember them, from my earliest recollections until my current age of 81. I will not guess at things I am not sure I remember, except that if they are interesting I will include them and indicate my uncertainties. Phyllis can describe my sleep patterns only since the time we met, when I had recently become 53, except that I am not sure how much I slept in the first years we bedded together.

After starting to write about some of my sleep experiences, I found the need to return here to write this one paragraph as a preface. In describing my own experiences, it occurred to me that I must describe my stages of life and some important circumstances that have affected my sleep patterns and habits. Without the accompanying causes, circumstances, and remedies, any description of my sleep patterns would not be very helpful to others, if not altogether meaningless. For these reasons, I have also convinced myself to shed some modesty and include feelings, circumstances, pressures, and stresses that have affected my sleep, which I had not initially been prepared to do. In any case, after listening to the sleep habits in college of some of our grandchildren, I do not think that any of the younger members of my family are likely yet to be concerned enough about their bad sleep patterns to pick up any book with a title including the word "insomnia."

I do not remember having any sleep problems that concerned me when I was in the age range of about 4 to 9 years old, although my parents might tell some if they were still here. I do remember having dreams at that early age. I remember one dream where I thought our home was burning and I was trapped in the basement. I let out a scream, and this awakened me.

Another dream that I seem to remember only vaguely is one in which I had walked in my sleep. I do not remember what age I was at the time, but I must have been a very young boy for this memory to be so vague. In this dream, I felt the need to get up and go to the toilet. I then got up, walked in my sleep, and urinated in the clothes closet. My great relief at this accomplishment immediately awakened me and I felt sorry for this dirty deed.

Other dreams I remember were dreams in which I could wave my arms in certain ways and fly up into the air like a bird. In these dreams I would tease my friends by throwing something at them (a snowball?) and then flying up out of range. Or, I would fly up into the air and spy into someone's window. I do not think I knew that was bad at that age, just mischievous and funny.

I do not remember being concerned as a child in my preschool years about any losses of sleep caused by these dreams. I was just happy to play or nap whenever the freedom to do so presented itself.

(Nowadays, I often wave my arms before playing tennis as part of my exercises, but I do not fly. I can't even jump more than an inch to hit a high lob. When my tennis friends see me doing my arm waves, they tell me I am having seizures. Anyhow, I am glad that as an octogenarian I can still stand up and walk on the courts, and on rare occasions shuffle over to intercept a cross-court shot without hitting it into the net.)

I do not remember having any sleep problems, or being sleepy in school in the elementary grades, or in the junior high years of seventh and eighth grades. I was just lackadaisical, absent minded, day-dreaming, and sometimes put into the cloakroom by the teacher for not paying attention or otherwise fooling around. I conclude that I must have had great teachers in the elementary and junior high grades, because I seemed to have learned enough of the basic ABCs to obtain high enough grades in the high eighth grade to be admitted early to the difficult "A course" at Baltimore Polytechnic Institute (Poly) in the ninth grade.

In the high eighth grade, and then in high school, where I became interested in improved academic and other performance, I began to realize the need for a certain amount of sleep. I tried in the high eighth grade to get much better grades only because my closest boyfriend, Josh Greenspon, whom I had known since kindergarten, kept bugging me to study enough to go to the same course at Poly that he was planning to enter. Josh was a more diligent student than I. Another friend, Al Viola, also came along with encouragement, as did a cousin, Arnold Brodsky, just before he went to Europe to serve in World War II. My mother questioned whether I could survive the hard work at Poly, having experienced so many problems with my earlier scholastic performance. My mother was afraid that I would need to stay up too late studying, not get enough sleep, and ruin my health. She cautioned me against enrolling in the A course at Poly, which had a reputation as the most difficult high school course in Baltimore.

However, I had an excellent algebra teacher in the high eighth grade, a Mr. Goldberg, and found that I could do well in math, surprising as it seemed. Doing some homework after dinner for a change, I began to find evening study often interesting and enjoyable. I have no recollection of being concerned about not having enough sleep in the early grades up to the eighth. If it had caused my inattentions in class, I did not know it. But now, with the desire to get at least an 80 in each course in order to be admitted to the Poly A course, I began to find that I sometime needed to sacrifice my hours of sleep in order to do well on tests the following day.

There were other experiences in the earlier ages of 12 or 13 that led me to follow my friend Josh's advice to pursue academic work. The first job I remember, other than painting baseboards for my paperhanger father for 25 cents a day as a child, was when I was employed to work in a grocery store one summer, doing odd jobs and delivering groceries on my small, non-coasting bike until I was exhausted. After only one week of work, Mr. Jablon, the grocer, fired me. I did not weigh out beans fast enough. I guess that I am not a good bean counter. Thus, I suspected that I would not be adept enough at simple tasks to support myself through life as a laborer or store helper, using my hands and tools. I would need some education so that I could someday work quietly at a desk, using only a pencil.

I was so lucky to have an early friend like Josh and an algebra teacher like Mr. Goldberg. I since have advised grandchildren to pick their friends and teachers carefully, and be lucky.

After I entered the ninth grade of Poly's A course in 1942 at age 13, my time for sleep was often limited. The A course was designed to provide about twice as much math instruction as well as other science and technical subjects relevant to an expected college engineering program. My daytime and most evening hours were well occupied with school, study, and sports practice, as well as three streetcar rides to and from school. On the streetcar rides, I did enjoy seeing some pretty girls, but I could not ask for dates in high school, and had no money for them if I did. For some relaxation, I often played piano or listened to music for a short time in the evenings. Wrestling and tennis practice, and team competitions during the Poly years tired me out in the afternoons, and added to the need for late-night study. I became revived somewhat after dinner by the increased intellectual challenges. I found that I could never meet the goal of 10 hours sleep each night that the wrestling coach made as a requirement. I was lucky to get even six or seven.

The intense evening study usually left me with a late surge of energy (a "second wind") around 10 to 11 P.M., so that it was tough to get to sleep even after I turned off lights and got into bed. So, I often would just close my eyes while waiting to go to sleep, and go over in my head the material I needed to remember for the next day.

One day in the term near the end of the eleventh year in Poly's A course, my fellow student in the aisle next to me, Sig Eckhaus, asked, "Are you going to take that scholarship test at Hopkins [*The* Johns Hopkins University (JHU)] next Saturday?" I had not known about this test, but was lucky to be asked. Poly's A course was designed to provide enough background that admission to the first year of engineering at JHU was possible without the need to take the senior high school year. As it turned out, I must have been feeling good the day of the scholarship test; I won a four-year scholarship that paid all tuition and fees, and also provided free used textbooks. Thus, I entered JHU in the fall of 1945, still only sixteen until the following November.

Another thing to tell grandchildren: Pick a desk in class that is next to a bright, savvy student, and get lucky again.

At JHU, I continued tryouts for wrestling and tennis, and also joined a fraternity and other activities to begin some social life. All of this again required taking three streetcars also to JHU, afternoons of tiring athletics, some meetings after classes, and a heavy load of difficult courses. Through the rest of my teens, late nights of study were again the rule rather than the exception. I made varsity wrestling and tennis teams in my first year at JHU, which also required trips and late nights of study. However, during the rest of college days, courses became even more difficult, and more late study was required without the athletic or much social activity. Yet, looking back, the Poly and Hopkins experiences were worth some loss of sleep. They led the way to a career in which most of my work required only pencils, paper, and computers. No shovels or tools were required.

Sleep loss often continued after I was graduated in engineering. I could not get a job as a chemical engineer that summer, except as a laboratory assistant for two graduate students, so I looked for a fellowship to graduate school. The only one available sent me to Oak Ridge, Tennessee, on an Atomic Energy Commission-National Research Council Fellowship in

Radiological Physics. Again, this fellowship required full-time study during the day, and I also took a night course to satisfy the math requirements for a Ph.D. in physics, which I thought I might later pursue. So again, little time for adequate sleep, if any social activity was to be enjoyed at all.

When I returned to the D.C. area to work at the Naval Research Laboratory in 1950, I got engaged and then married at age 22. This added additional obligations, in addition to a full-time job and some physics courses at night.

During the next 15 years, difficult jobs combined with evening as well as daytime graduate courses to advance my career required more late night study or writing, so I was usually exhausted by the time lights were turned out. During these years, I remember that I slept soundly for the six hours available. I remember that I was not aware of any dreams during this period. I did not worry about sleep loss because I needed to concentrate on what I had to do.

I finally finished another matriculation in graduate school at age 37, and I took no further courses during the night or day. However, I was promoted to a tenured Associate Professor at the University of Pittsburgh in 1966, and I still found, even without evening courses, the pressures to obtain research grants, mentor graduate students, travel around the nation on an epidemiological study, and write reports and papers was as taxing as my previous life. I found myself out of the frying pan and into the fire. Further positions after 1971, with evening teaching, continued the same time pressures that did not allow for more than about six hours of sleep. I was usually not able to get a good night's sleep until I retired from full-time employment at the age of 57.

Today, sleep experts advise that at least seven, preferably eight, and even more hours of sleep might be needed at my age to feel optimally energetic during the day. Sometimes, when I now get eight hours or more sleep, I do realize the benefits. I even walk better, with more bounce. However, even if I sleep less, I will still do what is needed or desired the next day, and take naps or wait for better sleep another time. I am now happy just to have the freedom to rest whenever I desire.

I learned early in life not to worry about sleep, but now am amazed that I am still alive and healthy at 81. Thus, I think that, if I am caused any small amount of sleep deprivation by Phyllis' night noises, they cannot be a real problem to me. I am just so happy that my energizer bunny is getting her needed rest.

I do not worry about being awakened, by Phyllis or any other cause. If I cannot return to sleep when I am awakened after two or three hours in the middle of the night, I usually lay quietly, resting and letting my mind wander as it may. If I do not drift back to sleep, very often my mind will wander in many directions to many topics. Sometimes my mind drifts to thoughts of friends or loved ones, current or in the past. Other times, I obtain some of my most important intuitive ideas on what I need to do the next day in work or fun activities.

If I have a problem that I want to solve, mathematical or otherwise, I think in the quiet of the night about all the factors involved and how they might be ordered or combined logically to solve the problem. Then, when I get to a computer or desk the next day, I often have an approach that, with more careful thought and logic, can lead to a solution useful in my teaching or research. (I am still teaching part time at Georgetown University and writing articles and books to share life experiences.)

I have found that others who have been involved in research or in developing new ideas, artwork, or products also think intuitively and creatively when they wake up too early. You will find in Chapter 6 that some of those who completed our questionnaires use wakeful hours at night to think creatively. The value of insights received during the quiet of night often tends to bring a feeling of euphoria at solving problems (similar to the joy of winning games). This euphoria sometimes compensates for any worries about sleep. These winning ideas and euphoria can make the next day's writing or other activities more productive.

Also, if after waking too early, I lay in bed peacefully without worrying but thinking quietly, I become rather rested by the time I need or want to arise. I then do not need to think about getting out of bed. Without thinking I autonomically get up and out of bed feeling energetic. If Phyllis is still asleep and I do not want to wake her, I just wait until my legs retract from the covers, throw them forward, and jump out of bed quietly without prior thought. Then, I put on my slippers and stealthily slip out of the bedroom.

I do remember reading in the *Baltimore Sun*, when I was still living with my parents, that some research had shown that only three hours of good sleep, if followed by relaxed and non-anxious rest in bed for about another five hours, was just about as good as eight hours of sleep. That is perhaps one early influence that has helped me avoid too much worry about sleep. Kornblatt,[1] as described toward the end of this chapter, has recently published a book on many naturopathic ways to relax and enjoy the hours of sleeplessness after waking, and reduce worry about sleep. However, she does not stress the value of creative thinking during the wakeful night.

In any case, to give another example, whether I get eight hours sleep, or return late from a meeting and wake up too early, on a nice day I will usually still get up to play tennis with my tennis buddies, exercise, and take a nap later if I need to. The day I wrote this paragraph, I had only four hours sleep the previous night, then drove early to the D.C.-Maryland area for an afternoon at the National Library of Medicine, followed by a late night dinner meeting. I left the dinner meeting in Bethesda, Maryland about 9:30 P.M., and with a rest stop and gas refill, arrived home at 1:30 A.M., falling asleep about 3 A.M. I got up at 6 A.M. to attend a course on Facebook social networking at Chesapeake College 85 miles back West, and arrived early in time for class. I left Chesapeake College at 12:30 P.M., needed a rest stop badly when I was within 50 miles of home, pulled over for a half-hour snooze, and arrived home at about 2:30 P.M. in the afternoon, just in time to meet an assistant in my home office and find some items to send to my tax accountant. Phyllis had left for a regional meeting of the Maryland Nurses Association, so there I was finishing two more pages of this section on my sleep patterns at 8:45 P.M., after only four hours sleep two nights before and three hours sleep the previous night. I did feel a bit light-headed and ready for a good night's sleep before the next morning's tennis. However, I did feel good about finishing a part of this write-up that Phyllis had been after me to complete; thus, I experienced the euphoria that I mentioned earlier. As noted by sleep authorities in some of our references, this kind of schedule should not be maintained for more than a couple of days. Yet, sometimes a certain amount of sleep loss can be paid for by the euphoria that can accompany needed, desired, or entertaining accomplishments.

The relief at finishing a job in time to meet a deadline that causes anxiety also leads to satisfaction and a release of tensions. If sleep time is urgently upon me, I must then counteract the effects of adrenalin, and then hope my body will release some endorphins through relaxed thoughts, some readings, dimmed lights, soft music, or other non-medical sleep assistance. Or, if it is not bedtime yet and more work or play is still ahead, closing my eyes and lying back to rest for ten minutes or more, or taking a short nap, will correct the situation.

My Life-Saving Discovery
to Avoid Falling Asleep While Driving

If I am driving at night after sleep loss and begin to feel sleepy, there are times when even loud music or an interesting radio program will not keep me awake. Sometimes I will stop at a safe location and take a short nap. However, toward the end of my trip home to Ocean Pines, Maryland, there are no convenient places to stop. I knew from previous experiences falling asleep at the wheel, only to have been saved by last-second wakenings, that I needed some special way to keep me awake at these times. I have for years practiced some of the songs I like, or written songs, to make long trips shorter, especially when I could not find intelligent life on earth by turning on the car radio. Finally, I discovered, a few years ago, that a great way to stay awake on the road is to choose a song where I need to use my entire range, in my case ending two octaves high above my lowest note. The exertion of throat muscles and vocal chords to sing the highest notes seems to send blood to my brain and bring me fully alert. I also sing as loudly as possible. I then become so wide awake that, even if I arrive home at 2 to 3 A.M. and want or need to arise after a few hours, I have trouble going to sleep. I need to stimulate my endorphins all over again. But at least, I have discovered that singing can save my life. I freely pass this discovery on to the readers of this book. If incorporated in driver training courses and added to safe driving recommendations, this discovery could save many lives that are currently lost from falling asleep at the wheel!

Also, an advantage that can be added by driving alone at night is that, whether one can carry a tune or not, if one wants to sing loudly, there are no complaints in a closed auto from anyone hearing the results.

How I Perceive That My Own Sleep Habits Affect Phyllis

In regard to how my sleep patterns or habits affect Phyllis, I have come to understand and accept her needs, and appreciate the differences between our natural biological clocks and circumstances. I try to adapt my habits to support her requirements for a more ordered life because I appreciate what a great partner she is and how she accomplishes tasks like an energizer bunny during the day if her sleep needs are met.

One problem I had until a few years ago was that she was disturbed by the noises I made because of the sleep apnea she told me I was exhibiting. As mentioned before, I lost 22 pounds by more exercise combined with the eating of fewer calories, in order to move faster on the tennis courts, in compensation for my slowing with age. Phyllis is no longer bothered by my sleep apnea, nor by my snoring as far as I know. I should also mention that I discovered in high school and college that a few hours of intense aerobic exercise also helped me sleep better at night, whenever I did not need to stay up too late studying.

Finally, if I get out of bed or go back into the bedroom while Phyllis is sleeping, I try to tiptoe quietly. Phyllis is one person who deserves, and well utilizes, a good night's sleep.

Summary of Allen's Sleep Habits

- Usually I go to bed by 9 to 11 P.M. and read in bed for an hour or two before turning out lights (wrong thing to do?). I would like to get up by 7 A.M. and perform like an energizer bunny, but often I get up feeling like an old man (I am) unless I combine at least three hours of sleep with restful or creative thinking in bed for another four or five hours. It seems that, following a few hours of good sleep, just being horizontal can provide a significant amount of the required physiologic restitution. This is my personal experience, confirming the *Baltimore Sun* article that I read years ago.

- Sometimes, if I am not feeling sleepy at bedtime, I will watch TV news or stories for an hour or two, in a living room out of the bedroom where Phyllis is sleeping (right thing to do).

- Sometimes, if falling asleep within 30 minutes or so, and sleeping for three or four hours before going to the bathroom, I feel refreshed, have a light breakfast at 3 or 4 A.M., and go up to my study to work for about two to three hours before going back to bed at 6 to 7 A.M.

- Sometimes, if I wake up after three or four hours, I just lie quietly resting and thinking freely as my mind wanders at random between subjects. This often allows the solving of problems intuitively and getting ideas for the next day's work or activities. On one of these mornings, I formulated a questionnaire and outline for this book, while Phyllis slept a few hours longer. I then was able to tell Phyllis when she awoke that I changed my mind and would join her as a co-author.

- My sleep pattern for any one night is unpredictable, but rarely do I get the eight hours or more of solid sleep I need to have optimum energy the next day. I usually need to take one or more naps, fifteen minutes or longer each, during the day to continue my planned tasks or activities.

- No matter how little sleep I get, I will arise at least by 8 A.M. if it is a good day for tennis. I will nap later, especially if I need energy to do my weight lifting or aerobic exercises after tennis. Forcing myself to exercise is almost impossible when I feel tired or lazy (which is often).

• I never worry that, because I have not had enough sleep, my health will fail, my work will not meet deadlines, or Phyllis will leave me. A long track record at this age makes me rather confident about the future.

Whether you call it insomnia or not, Allen's sleep habits are a mess. He just does not worry about insomnia, but if that is what he has, he lives with it. He looks forward to life and its interesting and enjoyable activities. Ask Phyllis.

A note about the book, *Restful Insomnia*: A few months after beginning to write this book, Phyllis and I bought a new book that provides a great number of suggestions for natural methods of living with insomnia without letting loss of sleep become an insurmountable problem. This book by Sondra Kornblatt suggests aspects of Allen's attitude toward sleep loss, and promises to help many persons who have insomnia but might not enjoy creative, relaxed thinking for dealing with insufficient sleep at night.[2] The creative thought practices described in our book are missing from Kornblatt's book. This does not detract from her accomplishment. Some of her more important suggestions are summarized later in this book.

General Observations About the Sleep Problems of Phyllis and Allen

It seems that between Phyllis and Allen, many or most of the sleep problems described by Neubauer as present for those perceiving and classified to have insomnia have been present to some degree in their adult lives.

As in the simple definition of Neubauer[3] adopted earlier, insomnia may be defined as: "Fundamentally, 'I have insomnia' means (1) 'I can't sleep' and (2) 'I'm suffering.'" Thus, I (Allen) do not worry about sleep loss. It does not usually affect my performance very much the next day, because I know that I can make up for sleep loss at a later time, or take naps the next day when the need becomes imperative. One of the main differences between Phyllis' sleep problems and mine is that I do not worry about sleep loss. Therefore, I do not suffer, and do not have insomnia.

We will see in Chapter 6 whether most or all of our sleep problems described in this chapter appear in the sample of persons who responded to our questionnaires. We will also see whether or not some additional insights are provided by the narratives based on these questionnaires.

CHAPTER 4

Sleep Patterns Throughout
the Life Cycle

Infancy

Immediately after birth, infants sleep about 16 to 20 hours during a 24-hour period, with wake periods to eat, to have their diapers changed, and to socialize, so to speak. Babies' circadian rhythms have not yet been established, so their wake periods when they choose to socialize can be at night. Babies generally don't have sleep problems; it's the parents who do, because they are awake when their newborns are. That's just how it is for awhile. It is indeed a difficult, although exciting, time for the parents. I remember my firstborn was initially up for an hour or so after he was fed. He was indeed "socializing." So we played with him, meaning we held him, and made funny noises and funny faces at him. He did indeed respond to us by alerting and beginning a subtle smile. As all parents, we were exhausted during the day, but that only lasted for three months—(it seemed more like an eternity). This is probably the most difficult part of adjusting to parenthood—losing sleep.

All three of my babies slept through the night (about six to seven hours) by three months of age. So did my grandbabies. My daughter, Beth-Ellen, gave birth to full-term twins when her firstborn was only 13 months old. Beth-Ellen was just chronically sleep deprived during those first few months of the twins' lives. So I believe three months is the magic number when newborns begin to sleep through the night, although it does vary.

According to Brazelton, about 70 percent of infants sleep about eight hours a night by three months of age; 83 percent sleep through by six months and 90 percent sleep through at about one year. Why is there such variance? Brazelton says some babies vary from normal sleep patterns due to premature birth and some variation is due to parental factors, such as reluctance to encourage independence—that is, letting the infant "work her way back to sleep." Doing so leads the infant toward self-comforting behaviors.[1] Light sleep cycles occur frequently during the night and are self-limiting. Generally, the infant can settle back down and fall into deep sleep, if not stimulated by the parent. Parents need to be taught to give the infant a chance to self-console herself. Otherwise, the baby will alert and "think" it is time to play and become conditioned to do so. Another reason infants awaken more at night is they are too docile and don't expend sufficient energy during the day. Hence they are more alert at night.[2]

However, Pantley, in her excellent book *The No Cry Sleep Solution* provides many ideas on gentle ways in which the parent can intervene without letting the baby just "cry it out."[3] Allen has used some of these techniques himself to help him and his former wife get adequate sleep when his three children were born, in the 1950s, and believes that Pantley is on the right track. An infant is not mean or contrary, and does not cry without reason. A parent's need for sleep can easily be accommodated by some of the techniques recommended by Pantley. Pantley's hero, Dr. William Sears, whose writings helped Pantley with her own infants, and who inspired her book, ends his foreword to her book with the paragraph: "At long last, I've found a book that I can hand to weary patients with the confidence that they can learn to help their baby sleep through the night—without the baby crying it out."[4]

Our personal experiences support the above references. Allen has often recalled how he managed to put each of the three children, of his first marriage of 32 years, to sleep without the need to let them cry for help. He believed at the beginning that newborns have no desire just to irritate their parents. They cry for good reasons, in order to communicate their specific needs. Because a newborn's stomach has capacity for only about an ounce of breast milk or formula, they have very little tolerance for gas bubbles. Their stomach capacity gradually increases as they grow.

Rather than lying the baby down to just cry to sleep, Allen would pick him up, cuddle him, dance with him, and give him enough firm pats on the back until some good burps released the gas bubbles. Then, Allen would lay the baby down on his tummy, massage his back gently, and sing to the baby a peaceful song, such as "I'll Be Loving You Always." (Allen's experience was in the 1950s, before it was known that it is important to place the baby on his or her back to sleep.) Repeating the song a number of times, each time more softly, combined with gentler and gentler back rubs, would eventually put a baby to sleep peacefully for a long time. In this way, Allen was able to lead each of his three infants into good sleep habits within a few weeks. It was necessary for Allen to assume this role at night, because his wife at the time was a teacher. Teachers need good sleep each night in order to do their best in the classroom.

Allen also has wondered whether the ignoring of a baby's need to burp when on her back might be a factor in the so-called mysterious sudden infant death syndrome (SIDS). When placing a baby on her back to sleep, you should then place a rolled up receiving blanket under her shoulder and back. The baby is then lying comfortably on her side if she spits up, and will not aspirate her milk.

We might refer to the advice given to Allen by Dr. Dankward Kodlin, a physician from Germany who became one of Allen's professors of biostatistics at the University of Pittsburgh in the early 1960s, about the need for adults to avoid suffocation from gastric reflux of their own food eaten late at night. Dr. Kodlin believed that many who were indicated on death certificates as having died of heart failure were actually victims of gastric reflux of food eaten soon before going to bed, without adequate digestion or raising their heads in the bed. The food refluxed was then thought to enter the trachea and suffocate the victim.

Even if having eaten about two hours before going to bed, Allen often still has heartburn, especially after eating too spicy or too fatty of foods, and needs to have his ice-cream soda before going to bed. (He gave up on Alka-Seltzers or other OTC medications, because he found that ice-cream sodas always worked and tasted much better.) He also, before lying down, punches his abdomen firmly a number of times until digestive gases are burped away. He then lies down on two pillows to raise his head a bit, and soon turns to one side or the other to go to sleep. If he does not read too long in bed, he often can then go to sleep soundly for a number of hours sufficient to refresh his energy. Of course, an infant cannot put pillows under her head, or go to the refrigerator to make an ice-cream soda after her parents go to sleep. Nor can she pat herself on the back or sing to herself.

Phyllis also had successful experiences leading her children into pleasant sleeping patterns within the first few months after birth. She would pick them up, cuddle them, and breastfeed them, usually not needing to let them "cry it out." In her years as a clinical and childbirth instructor, Phyllis has taught parents the importance of cuddling and soothing a baby, and then putting him down to sleep on his back in a calm, quiet room conducive to sleep. She has taught parents to pick up the baby if he continues to cry, because he likely needs another final burp in order to go back to sleep.

Thus, both Phyllis' and my experiences are consistent with those of Pantley. We highly recommend obtaining a copy of her book for use throughout the early stages of your child's life. Only a personal copy of Pantley's book will provide all of the tools for use in adopting her methods.

I (Phyllis) believe that some infants just innately aren't great sleepers. Talking to many women through the years, I have learned that some babies don't sleep through the night until they are much older. Sometimes there are good reasons (which I will address shortly) and sometimes parents have done everything right, but their babies still need to be fed or attended to at night. That's what parenthood is all about, and most of us adjust to it, get some sleep when we are able to, and begin to recoup when our babies begin to extend their sleep hours during the night.

Some babies don't even sleep through the night as late as two years old. According to Coren, parents of newborns lose about 400 to 750 hours of sleep during the first year after the baby's birth, usually averaging about two hours per night until their baby is four or five months of age. Additionally, the parents' sleep is fragmented and non-restorative, all leading to a large sleep debt.[5] Coren estimated that seven hours of fragmented sleep is equivalent to five-and-one-half hours of continuous sleep in regards to the ability to function mentally. Coren's book provides a simple list of "Twelve Tips for Sleepy Parents and Sleepless Children," as well as much detailed information on matters of sleep at all ages for those who wish to delve further on the scientific studies of causes and effects of sleeplessness.[6]

As indicated before, most parents survive this large sleep deficit and carry on. There are some mothers who do have postpartum depression. Loss of sleep isn't the cause of this, but it doesn't help the situation. However, that topic is another book in itself.

As we have learned in the previous chapters, normal circadian rhythms are governed by light and darkness. This takes some time to develop in newborn infants. They lived in darkness for nine months and did quite a bit of sleeping during that time. I was a previous maternal-newborn nurse and educator. When I attended women in labor and they were hooked up to a fetal monitor, there were definite wave patterns of the fetal heart rate that indicated when the fetus was sleeping. Newborns' sleep-awake cycles are governed by their needs to eat, and to be changed, cuddled, and nurtured. This includes "play" time to encourage socialization. Newborns do respond to attention from their caregivers. This stimulation is so important for brain development—cognitive and physical growth.

On the average, newborns' sleep cycles are about 50 to 60 minutes, contrasting with the adult cycle of 90 minutes. When newborns fall asleep, they go directly into REM sleep, referred to in the newborn as "active" sleep.[7] This means they move their arms and legs, make funny faces, grimace, and even appear to smile. They also startle easily, by flinging out their arms, then bringing them back toward their bodies. If you look closely at a newborn during this stage of sleep, you can observe his or her eyes moving under the eyelids. Apparently, the paralysis that accompanies REM sleep in adults does not happen in infants.

Do newborns dream? It is theorized that dreams occupy about half of infants' sleep time during a 24-hour day and that dreams are necessary for brain development. According to Dement, "dreaming is a form of awareness, an ability to put together sensory information and thoughts in a way that mimics what happens when we are awake."[8]

Infants spend long hours in deep sleep. In this stage, they are unresponsive to sound, light, touch, or heat stimuli. They have shorter periods of "ultradian" cycles, which are sleep periods that last between one and two hours followed by brief periods of wakefulness. This cycle changes to about four-hour rhythms by the time they are about two to eight weeks old.[9] According to Dement, infants' homeostatic drive leads to a buildup of sleep debt over a few hours and they "pay it back right away with a nap."[10]

Infants' sleeping patterns begin to stabilize between three months and one year of age, a blessing for the parents who can then obtain more uninterrupted sleep and have more energy during the day.

By six months, infants' biological clocks are well enough developed that most of them sleep at night without the need for feeding, if they are well fed during the day. By nine months, between 70 to 80 percent of infants sleep about nine to twelve hours through the night.[11] Infants will continue to take naps during the day. Before long they will have more predictable schedules, such as taking morning and afternoon naps for one or more hours. The length of the nap is very variable among infants. Eventually, they will take one long nap (hopefully) during the day.

Rosen's article, a more recent review of 48 peer-reviewed articles selected from examination of 161 articles as pertinent to her study, indicates that some of the above findings require further interpretation.[12] Studies using actigraphy (video observations of the infant through the night) provide information not available from interviews of the parents or any notes they have made. Videos indicated that quiet infant awakenings during the night were not recognized by parents whose sleep was not disrupted. Forty-four percent of two-month-olds and 78 percent of nine-month-olds (similar to Stores' finding above) were reported by parents to sleep through the night, whereas video recordings showed that only 15 percent of two-month-olds and 33 percent of nine-month-olds actually slept through the night without any wakeful moments.

Rosen also found in the literature that sleep patterns can be detected in utero at the same time as gestation is visible. (This corresponds to my [Phyllis'] observations as an obstetric nurse many years ago, as described above.) Sleep stages and cycles have been identified at 35 weeks after conception, but are not fully developed until about six months after birth. Circadian rhythms are disorganized for the first few weeks of life, with about equal amounts of sleep time during the day and during the night. At about two months, night sleep begins to dominate. The circadian-driven hormones melatonin and cortisol are not endogenously produced until three months of age.

T. Berry Brazelton, M.D., pediatrician and internationally known expert on child development, in his book, *Touchpoints*, suggested the following techniques for parents to help guide their babies into independent, self-comforting measures to go to sleep:

• Institute a relaxing, calm and nurturing routine at bedtime.
• Don't put her to sleep in your arms or while breastfeeding. Instead, put her in her crib, sit awhile to help her learn her own pattern or pat her soothingly.
• Wake her before your own bedtime for feeding, talk to her lovingly, hug her, and then repeat the first two techniques.
• Reinforce a particular "lovey"—a blanket, stuffed animal, or doll.
• Expect her to arouse and cry out about every three to four hours, such as 10 P.M., 2 A.M., and 6 A.M. Instead of taking her out of the crib, soothe, stroke or pat her gently.
• After a while, don't go to her, just talk to her soothingly outside of her room, and reassure her that she can do it on her own.[13]

These recommendations of Brazelton's come from a physician of long experience. However, those with newborns would also do well to examine the later behavioral recommendations in Pantley's book. The even later 2008 article by Rosen further supports Pantley's "No Cry Sleep Solution" approach.[14] Rosen, a nurse completing her doctoral dissertation, cautions against following statements in the literature and from the NIH that recommend always placing the baby down to sleep in a separate bed and avoidance of bed sharing. She recognizes, as found by Pantley, that with proper conditions, bed nursing and sharing can have long-term benefits to both mother and child. Her recommendations for safe bed sharing, in Table 2 of her article, are very similar to those recommended in Pantley's earlier book. Also, most of the literature Rosen reviewed points to the fact that recommendations regarding bed sharing are not dependent upon whether the infant is being fed by breast or bottle.

Babies should be put down to sleep when they show signs of sleepiness: beginning signs of irritability, rubbing their eyes, fussing or beginning to cry, when we know they have been well fed. At the time of this writing, I (Phyllis) have a ten-month-old great-grandbaby. When I spend time with my great-grandbaby, her sleepy behaviors are typical. The great-grandbaby has a very pleasant disposition and rarely cries. When she is tired and sleepy, she "complains," rubs her eyes, squirms when you try to hold her, and is very restless.

When signs of sleepiness, such as these, are observed, it is time to go through the bedtime (or naptime) ritual, as suggested by Dr. Brazelton, or by Pantley. Babies will soon learn to soothe themselves and go to sleep independently. Of course, make sure their hunger is satisfied first, and they are changed (and bathed if this is the nighttime ritual).

Coren further suggests that parents should establish a regular and predictable ritual associated with sleep, such as bathing, feeding, putting on pajamas, softly singing a lullaby, and when they are a little older, reading or telling a bedtime story. Also, turn on a night-light so the baby can see familiar objects in the room, but dim enough to stimulate secretion of melatonin. "Darkness is often equivalent in the child's mind to abandonment."[15] Pantley provides further support for these methods.

Toddlers and Young Children

By one year of age, babies need about 12 to 14 hours of sleep in a 24-hour period. The good part is that their longest sleep periods shift to night with two daytime naps. By 18 months of age, naps may decrease to once during the day and last about one to three hours. It is a good idea not to let the child nap too close to bedtime. Children may resist going to bed; fears and nightmares are common in this age group. Increased motor, cognitive, and social skills are competing forces against sleep time. Also, separation anxiety and development of imagination can cause some sleep problems. Daytime sleepiness, irritability and behavior problems can signal sleep deficit.[16]

By the age of two years, children generally have few nighttime awakenings. About five percent of this age group continues to awaken a few times a night. Science has not yet established how much sleep toddlers and young children need. Sleep debt is expressed differently in children than in adults. Although children may appear sleepy, they are more likely to become hyperactive and impulsive, have wide emotional swings, and have poor social relations with other children.[17]

Some of the reasons young children do not get sufficient sleep and develop sleep debt is because they have poor sleep hygiene—they don't have a regular bedtime schedule according to their needs, there may be too much noise and light in their room environment, and they possibly engage in over-stimulating activity prior to bedtime. Emotional and stress factors may also play a role in the cause of children's sleep problems.[18]

Sleep problems are common in toddlers and young children. They frequently resist going to sleep at expected times or they wake up during the night wanting something (such as a drink of water) to get attention from their parents. They sometimes wake up crying, fearful of being alone. Nightmares and night terrors are common in this age group.[19]

Dement cites Dr. Richard Ferber, a pediatrician and expert on children's sleep problems. Dr. Ferber advocates behavioral conditioning from six months of age on. His suggestions are similar to Dr. Brazelton's in that the parents should go into the child's room and verbally reassure him, but not physically comfort—pick up and hold—or feed him. If the child continues to cry, the parent should go back in five minutes and repeat the ritual. The next time wait 10 minutes, then 15, and so on.[20]

When children are awake and active, they are adamantly opposed to sleeping and don't feel sleepy as long as they are active and busy. But when they are ready for sleep, there is little parents or caretakers can do to stop them. The homeostatic sleep drive is so strong in young children that even strong stimuli do not trigger full wakefulness. This fact contributes to night terrors and sleepwalking. (These will be discussed in Chapter 7.) Occasional nightmares are common and can be genuinely frightening experiences, so it is important for parents to comfort and reassure the child during these episodes. Like adults, children have different sleep needs. Once parents establish how much their children need they should establish a bedtime routine and ritual and stick to it. Delaying children's bedtime by as little as a half-hour can have profound effects. Dement attributes much of children's behavioral and learning problems to insufficient sleep at night.[21]

Some children do have sleep problems that they don't outgrow; such problems can continue for years if untreated. The negative impact of sleep deficit in the child can also disrupt the sleep of the family. Children's sleep problems can be the result of biological and psychological influences. Some common sleep disturbances in children include bedtime resistance, night waking, nightmares, and sleep terrors. (These will further be described in Chapter 7.) Children's sleep difficulties can also be associated with more complex and less common disorders, such as sleep apnea and restless leg syndrome (covered in the next chapter). Bedtime disturbances and night waking occur in about 40 percent of infants and 25 to 50 percent of preschoolers.[22]

Durand and his associates conceptualized children's sleep disorders on two integrated perspectives. The first assumption is that some children are biologically vulnerable to sleep disturbances. Psychological factors also play a role. The second assumption is that these vulnerabilities are reinforced by the parents' actions in trying to settle their children down for sleep. "In other words, personality characteristics sleep difficulties, and parental reactions interact in a reciprocal manner to produce and maintain sleep problems."[23] Children's sleep disturbances should be medically evaluated and treated by qualified medical practitioners specializing in children's sleep disorders. Interventions are individualized according to the disturbance. For example, a combination of interventions has been approached, including establishing bedtime routines and graduated extinction.[24]

In her book, *Insomniac*, Gayle Green relates her problems of insomnia, which, she says, began in infancy. She discovered letters that her mother wrote to her father after he was drafted in World War II. Her mother wrote in March 1944 how Gayle, then 18 months old, hated to go to sleep. There were many letters, up until October 1945, describing how Gayle stayed up in her crib for hours before finally falling asleep.[25] Green contends that "human beings are born with different sleep propensities." Some people sleep well; others are hyperalert. Homeostatic and circadian systems vary among people, suggesting that sleep patterns are "genetically defined."[26]

I tend to agree with this analysis. When you talk to enough people, you learn that there is a wide variance in how much sleep people need and how well some folks function with less than required sleep for the particular age group. This goes for young children as well.

School-Aged Children

Infants' and toddlers' poor sleep habits often continue into childhood. Although there is no conclusive scientific evidence, it is believed that children who have sleep disturbances continue to have them throughout adulthood.[27] Some of the same reasons underlying sleep disturbances in toddlers apply to children as they grow older, such as over-stimulation prior to bedtime, fears, stresses, and nightmares. Also, bedtime may be set too early for some children who are just not sleepy at the time their parents set. Children who engage in stimulating activities, such as active playing and running around will become aroused. Also watching an action-packed movie or TV program will work against promoting a calm environment that is conducive for sleep at bedtime.

Children ages five to twelve years need about ten to eleven hours of sleep at night. Desired activities, interests, and schoolwork may conflict with getting to bed early enough to obtain sufficient hours of needed sleep. With ever-expanding technology, such as video games, iPods, cell phones, and so many more, early sleep is not a priority for many children, particularly if these items are in the child's bedroom. In addition, drinking caffeinated beverages, such as cola, too close to bedtime can cause arousal instead of sleepiness.[28]

Fifteen to 27 percent of school-aged children resist going to bed. These percentages increase in children with special needs. For example, children with attention deficit hyperactivity disorder (ADHD)—a disorder in which children exhibit hyperactivity, impulsiveness, and inattention—display difficulty initiating and maintaining sleep. Up to 80 percent of children with other developmental disorders, including autism, suffer from inability to initiate and maintain sleep. Poor or inadequate sleep leads to mood swings, behavioral problems, poor schoolwork, and hyperactivity. There are more cases of ADHD in recent years. Dement questions if some of these children are really just sleepy.[29]

After I retired, I did some school nursing for a few years in an intermediate school (grades 4 to 6). It really surprised me to see how many children were taking medications for ADHD or ADD. The medications for these disorders are actually stimulants that have the opposite effects on children with ADHD or ADD than on adults. Such medications have a stimulating effect on adults but decrease the hyperactive and distractibility symptoms of ADHD in children. However, many of the children that came for their medication in the health office at school rebelled against taking these medications, because they complained of difficulty sleeping at night.

Researchers have found connections between childhood-onset insomnia and dyslexia and ADHD. Such children have difficulty focusing, concentrating, sitting still, and controlling their emotions, all of which can affect learning. The disorder begins in childhood and sometimes continues into adulthood. The overall prevalence of ADHD is four to five percent and is more prevalent in boys than in girls. The disorder is linked with a variety of sleep problems. According to a 2004 National Sleep Foundation in America poll, more than two-thirds of children have one or more sleep problems at least a few nights a week. Children who have been diagnosed with ADHD have higher rates of daytime sleepiness than children who do not have this disorder. Other research has shown that 50 percent of children with ADHD had symptoms of sleep disordered breathing. If sleep problems are an issue, treating these problems may improve symptoms of ADHD.[30] Children who have insomnia may also have underlying medical or emotional disturbances. Some children have obstructed sleep apnea (OSA), which is much more common in adults. In children, it is generally due to enlarged tonsils and adenoids, which greatly narrows the airway passage in the back of the throat. This causes the child to stop breathing (apnea) and briefly wake up. This happens many times throughout the night, thereby preventing uninterrupted, restorative sleep. This problem is covered in greater detail, along with other underlying conditions that cause insomnia, in Chapter 5. The major symptom of OSA in children is snoring. If the child is snoring, it is important for parents to observe their child while he or she is sleeping, to listen for snoring and observe carefully for periods of apnea (absence of breathing). This condition should be corrected promptly. It is also fairly common for children to have nightmares, night terrors, sleep talking and sleepwalking. These conditions are discussed thoroughly in Chapter 7.

Although rare, true (also called idiopathic or primary) insomnia does begin in childhood. Gayle Green, in her book *Insomniac*, discussed research conducted on childhood-onset insomnia by Hauri and Olmstead. These authors hypothesized that true insomnia is not caused by psychopathological factors, but instead has an underlying neurophysiologic and neurochemical basis. This means there is an impairment in the sleep center of the brain.[31] Much of Green's book is autobiographical. She has had insomnia since she was a very young child.

Many of these children also have strong reactions to certain foods and caffeinated beverages. Other causes of childhood-onset insomnia could be extreme sensitivity to environmental stimulation, such as noise, and to atypical reactions to certain medications.[32] There does seem to be a genetic connection to childhood-onset insomnia, as some studies have shown. Mothers are the most frequently afflicted. According to Green, "[A]necdotal evidence suggests that insomniac parents have insomniac children, and insomniac children have insomniac parents."[33]

Adolescence

Dement describes adolescence perfectly. "When puberty strikes, the hormones rage, the heart beats faster, and parents' blood pressures rise." It is these raging hormones that rewire the brain, particularly the cerebral cortex. "The scale of the changes during puberty is unmatched again until very old age...."[34] The sex hormones—testosterone, follicle-stimulating hormone, and leutenizing hormone—are all released mainly during sleep, having an impact on the sleep cycle during puberty. Melatonin also plays an important role in maturation during adolescence. Decreased levels of melatonin signal the beginning of puberty. If levels stay high, puberty will be delayed.[35]

The adolescent brain undergoes profound biological transformations.

There is a precipitous (about 40 percent) decline in the deepest sleep stage (fourth stage). Prior to menstruation, the prevalence of adolescent insomnia is about the same for boys and girls, but is about two and a half times greater in girls following menstruation.[36] Estrogen triggers the release of cortisol, which in turn, triggers arousal and the stress response.

Teens still need about nine or more hours of sleep at night, just about the same amount needed at younger childhood ages. However, most teens don't get enough sleep. Teens' biological clocks undergo significant change, so that many teens don't feel sleepy in the evening. Their circadian timing system seems to slow down, so their initial sleep phase is delayed.[37] This "delayed-phase syndrome" is one of the underlying causes of insomnia described in the next chapter. The problem is that they have to get up earlier than their natural arousal time to get to school on time.

One school in Edina, Minnesota, referred to as the "Minnesota project," did change school start time from 7:20 to 8:30 A.M. As a result, "district officials reported that students were far more awake and engaged in class, and the number of behavioral problems went down."[38]

In addition to their biological clocks adjusting, adolescents choose to stay up much later than they should because of more desirable competing activities, such as watching their favorite TV programs, communicating with friends via email, text messaging, and engaging in other technological and media advances. Many teens have televisions and other "tech" equipment in their bedrooms. Parents are probably long asleep while their teens are busy at whatever they are doing, when they should be sleeping. Another necessity—although not as interesting as these activities—is homework that must in some way get done, usually at the expense of much needed sleep. Moreover, teens are known to drink lots of sodas, which are chock full of caffeine and sugar, all of which triggers cortisol secretion, which leads to a state of arousal.

Adolescents are more impaired by sleep loss than adults. Sleep deficit affects learning and is related to increase in aggression and violence, and use of drugs. Furthermore, sleep deficit can lead to chronic sleep disorders. There is current evidence that teens are extremely sleep-deprived. They build up a sizable sleep debt. As a result they experience decreased alertness, poor school performance, and decreased memory and problem-solving skills. Once teens get to sleep, they sleep soundly and it is extremely difficult to wake them up in the morning in time to get ready for school.[39]

Chronic sleep deficit can also have an effect on normal body growth and tissue repair, as explained in Chapter 2. A major hormone, secreted by the pituitary gland, is growth hormone (GH). The release of this hormone is facilitated by growth hormone releasing factor (GHRF), secreted in the hypothalamus (which houses the sleep center of the brain). These important hormones are responsible for growth and tissue repair from infancy through teenhood. After growth ceases, GH is still secreted in lesser amounts throughout life as necessary for tissue repair. Throughout life, higher concentrations of these hormones are secreted during deep, slow-wave sleep (stages 3 and 4) than during other sleep stages or at other times. This is just one of the major reasons that children and teens should get their required amount of sleep.

What can be done about remedying teens' sleep deficits? Any parents trying to cope with all the idiosyncrasies of their adolescent children probably throw up their hands and roll their eyes in perplexity and frustration. One solution could be to start school classes later. This would be very complicated and take much coordination and effort. Parents should educate their teen children about the importance of adequate sleep, encourage them to practice good sleep hygiene, keep their tech and game equipment in a room other than their bedroom, and discourage caffeinated beverages in the afternoon and evening hours.

My grandson, David, is 21 years old and just graduated from a nearby university. He has come here to visit regularly and had lived here for a couple of months during the summer prior to attending the university. So I'm fairly familiar with his sleep habits, which are typical of present-day teens and young adults. He usually doesn't go to sleep until very late—between 12 and 2 A.M.—in my estimation. He has told me it is not a problem; it is because his "body clock" doesn't tell him he is sleepy until late in the evening and because of homework that had to be done. Sometimes he goes to bed even later if he is out socializing with friends, which certainly is part of university life. He sometimes reads or watches television before turning off the lights. He does not wake in the night once asleep, although he does have trouble falling asleep if he has a lot of schoolwork to do, relationship issues or other stresses. If he can't get enough sleep, he does feel drowsy, tired, and not alert. He still claims he does not have any sleep problems.

I (Phyllis) have enjoyed my grandson's visits and have tried (in vain) to lovingly "teach him" to take good care of himself—to eat healthy, to dress warm in cold weather, to drive safely, and to get enough sleep. I hope some of it will sink in. He is an adult now and makes his own decisions. He is motivated and strives for good grades. He is now getting ready to attend graduate school.

Teens and young adults have to find their own ways, and hopefully, make the right choices. Just as in young children, true insomnia does affect a small percentage of children, teens, and young adults. They should seek medical attention, be evaluated for underlying physical or psychological causes or for idiopathic insomnia, and be treated to best meet their needs.

Adulthood

Biological changes in our bodies and brains continue throughout adulthood and into old age. According to Dement, shortly after our early 20s, "our bodies start the slow process of falling apart." "[T]he muscles lose strength and mass. We begin to gain fat. Our skin begins to lose resiliency and firmness."[40] This is just what we want to hear, right? But these are the facts of life. Of course, such changes do not occur in all people at the same chronological age. There are both intrinsic and environmental factors that affect our health, continued development, and sleep patterns.

Part of this picture includes changes in sleep architecture, which refers to the 90-minute sleep cycle—the order of the sleep stages and how long each stage of sleep lasts. Changes in sleep architecture through the life cycle are due to biological and maturational factors. Just as there are other physical changes that occur with age, sleep patterns also change. Some people have a more difficult time falling asleep and/or staying asleep. It is not just amount of sleep that people actually get that affects well being, but also the quality of sleep.

The most profound change that occurs as we get older is the time spent in delta (slow-wave) sleep, the deepest stage of the sleep cycle. A twenty-year-old person gets, on the average, 45 minutes or so of delta sleep each night, mostly during the first few hours of sleep. However, by age sixty, the amount of time spent in delta sleep is greatly reduced.[41] The amount of sleep needed as we age is a mystery. Experts have differing views on this. One study of a large sample of middle-aged adults (aged 40 to 65 years) showed an average amount of sleep was seven hours per night.[42] According to Schenck, about 16 percent of adults get less than six hours of sleep per night.[43]

The results from a large meta-analysis of 65 different studies showed the changes in sleep architecture that occur from age 5 through old age. The authors concluded that sleep latency (the time it takes to fall asleep) and sleep stages 1 and 2 increase with age. REM sleep time increases from childhood to adolescence, then decreases with age in adults. After adolescence, the percentage of REM sleep remains stable until after 60 years of age, when time spent in REM sleep begins to decline. Results also showed that adults' total sleep time, sleep efficiency (ratio of total sleep to time spent in bed), the percentage of slow-wave (deep) sleep, of REM sleep, and REM latency all consistently decrease with age.[44]

In another study, researchers sought to determine changes in the percentage of REM sleep through the life cycle. Their findings showed variations between and within results of other research reported in the literature. The authors seemed to prefer the finding that the amount of REM sleep decreases about 0.6 percent per decade. Why should this be important to know? The authors explain "that REM sleep is involved in perceptual learning, memory consolidation, synthesis of new information, or arrangement of information into a network of internal association."[45] If significant, this could explain, in part, why there is some decline in mental functioning in some people of advanced age. However, the variations in findings within the literature, and the very small percent per decade indicated by Floyd et al., followed in some cases with increases in percent per decade in the 70 age group, put the conclusions of Floyd et al. in considerable doubt. We (AB and PLB) are not convinced about the conclusion that a decrease in REM sleep with age in older adults is a reason for diminished memory. Nor do we believe that our amounts of REM sleep have any effect at all on our memory capacities.

There is much research evidence that insomnia affects more women than men. It is possible that more women complain and worry about sleep difficulties than men do. I (Phyllis) certainly complain more about my sleep problems much more than my husband does (as you've probably surmised from the authors' stories in Chapter 3). It's those female hormones that play a large role in women's sleep disturbances. Of course, through the ages women's physical and mental disorders have been blamed on their reproductive systems. However, female hormones (estrogen and progesterone) do play a major role underlying women's sleep disturbances. The female hormone estrogen does stimulate cortisol, as stated earlier, which is the "alerting" hormone. So there is a physiologic reason for this occurrence.

It is well documented that following puberty, the fluctuations of female hormones surrounding the menstrual cycle, pregnancy, postpartum, and menopause do have an effect on women's sleep patterns. Such hormonal fluctuations affect many systems in the body and mediate other hormonal systems in the brain and body. This includes regulation of the biological clock, and so also affects the quality of sleep. I am not saying that all women in their reproductive years are vulnerable to sleep disorders. Some women are more vulnerable to these hormonal fluctuations than others. From adolescence through women's reproductive years, menstrual symptoms, such as bloating, cramping, and mood changes, can deter sleep. Premenstrual syndrome (PMS) is an intensification of these symptoms, which are very disturbing and can cause further sleep difficulties.

Estrogen levels are highest in the days before and during ovulation, a time when REM sleep also increases slightly. Progesterone levels increase following ovulation and body temperature rises slightly. Both hormones are at their lowest levels prior to the onset of menstruation. Women tend to complain of restlessness, difficulty falling asleep, and poor sleep quality during this time of the cycle.[46] Sleep problems can be exacerbated if women have pre-menstrual syndrome (PMS), severe cramping and bloating during menstruation, or other menstrual dysfunctions. Any discomfort or mood disorders obviously affect sleep. When menstrual-related symptoms are treated, sleep problems are likely to be abated.

Pregnancy is another difficult time for women in regard to sleep. Women's so-called discomforts of pregnancy can occur throughout the ten lunar months. During the first trimester (first three months), women can experience morning sickness, fatigue, breast tenderness and frequent urination. Such symptoms can be severe, very mild or even non-existent. Any of these symptoms can disrupt sleep. Some women have severe nausea that extends well beyond the first trimester. During the second trimester, discomforts that can disturb sleep include pressure on the urinary bladder and on muscles and ligaments, heartburn, shortness of breath, leg cramps, and restlessness due to the enlarging uterus. These symptoms also are due to the hormones, particularly progesterone, which causes relaxation of muscles and joints. The same symptoms progress into the third trimester and worsen due to the enlarging uterus. Add to this the baby's movements, particularly disturbing at night when the woman is trying to sleep.

Many pregnant women have serious sleep problems, and frequently doctors are unaware of the serious health problems that can result. A 1998 National Sleep Foundation poll found that 80 percent of women reported disturbed sleep during pregnancy.[47] Increased progesterone levels are also responsible for nasal congestion. Some women begin to snore and might even be troubled with sleep apnea (described in detail in the next chapter). Also, some women may experience restless leg syndrome (RLS) (also in next chapter), a very disturbing uncontrollable urge to move their legs in response to tingling and other unpleasant sensations in their legs.[48]

Pregnancy can be a stressful time in women's lives. In addition to the physical discomforts mentioned above, women certainly have concerns about the health of their unborn babies, their own health, work-related fatigue, relationships, and other concerns that may plague anyone at any time. If there are relational, social, financial, or other emotional issues, these factors are also likely to further contribute to sleep disturbances. Addressing these problems could help relieve sleep difficulties.

There are several ways to relieve physical discomforts, such as eating small, frequent, light meals; drinking lots of fluids (water, milk, juices) between meals; not lying down after a meal; and avoiding fried and spicy foods. When going to sleep, it is helpful to use lots of pillows—placing one between her legs, one behind to support her back, one in front to support her abdomen, and one under her head. Other comfort measures can be found in the myriad of books on pregnancy. Other existing medical or other underlying sleep problems, such as sleep apnea or RLS, should be treated. Pregnant women should not take hypnotic or over-the-counter medications. They should also avoid consuming any alcoholic beverages or caffeinated beverages. One cup of coffee or tea in the morning is safe.

Women, of course, have trouble sleeping after the baby is born, mainly because newborn babies do not have a circadian rhythm as yet—and they need to be fed every couple of hours. Many women suffer from fatigue from loss of sleep due to discomfort during the last month of pregnancy and during labor. So they are already sleep deprived. Insomnia is not the problem, but sleep deficit is. Babies' circadian rhythms are not established until they are about three or more months of age. Parents are going to be sleep deprived until this happens. The best advice I've given to parents is to sleep when the baby sleeps, day and night, and limit visitors to a minimum. If family members and friends do come to visit, don't entertain them—you are the one who needs pampering. Just put them—mom, dad, sister, whoever—to work. (I taught childbirth education classes for many years and advocated these measures.)

To further complicate the sleep deficit of new mothers, about three to five days after birth, many women experience postpartum blues. Symptoms include a "let-down" feeling and sadness. About 75 to 80 percent of postpartum women experience these symptoms, which are basically due to the profound drop in hormones secreted by the placenta, particularly progesterone and estrogen. The blues are typically confined to the first week after the baby is born.[49] Fatigue, due to sleep deprivation and new mothering responsibilities, also plays a role in causing the "blues." These "blues" are quite normal, but still can be disturbing.

However, if the "blues" persist and become more severe, they may be symptomatic of postpartum depression. This is not normal, so it is imperative that the woman seek medical attention. Symptoms of postpartum depression include severe sadness, insomnia, fatigue, inability to perform daily activities and care of baby. This condition is not so uncommon as previously thought to be. There are antidepressive medications that are effective and do not affect breastfeeding. Depression is one underlying cause of insomnia.

There are other factors involved besides hormonal fluctuations that affect women's sleep patterns. Since women began entering the work force in greater numbers since the second half of the twentieth century, the added burdens and time necessary to juggle occupational and family responsibilities has left less time for sufficient and restful sleep. Additionally, certain chronic conditions that are more prevalent in women affect the restorative sleep quality. These conditions include fibromyalgia, chronic fatigue syndrome, osteoarthritis, depression, and the occurrence of stressful life events, such as intimate partner violence or other family crises.[50]

Middle Aged

The term "middle age" conjures up thoughts of "we're over the hill" in some women. I (Phyllis) believe the definitions of this period in our lives have changed in modern times. At one time 40 years of age was considered "old." Now 40-year-olds seem so young to me. My own daughters and son have surpassed this young age. No matter how we feel, it is a fact that our bodies continue to change throughout the life span. However, all people's bodies and brains do not change at the same time and so "aging" health problems cannot be generalized to specific chronologic ages. When we consider change, we look at women's biological changes, rather than men's, because, in women, there is a definite marker. It is called menopause, which is a time in the life span when female hormones are gradually diminished and the menstrual cycle ceases. Men can also have biological issues that disturb their sleep (again discussed in the next chapter), but women have more problems with insomnia that are related to their hormonal changes during this time in their lives.

Results from research studies have shown that about 50 percent of women have various sleep disturbances when they enter menopause.[51] When a woman's menstrual period changes, prior to complete cessation of menses, that period of time is referred to as "premenopause." Menopause is the complete cessation of menses. At the same time that this occurs, the ovaries stop producing eggs and the production of estrogen and progesterone are gradually decreased. However, the adrenal glands continue to secrete some estrogen. "Perimenopause" is a term used to describe symptoms prior to menopause, during menopause, and post-menopause.

Estrogen and progesterone, secreted during women's reproductive years, are necessary for purposes of fertility and secondary sexual characteristics. Decreasing levels of these hormones cause perimenopausal symptoms that can disrupt restorative sleep. These symptoms can begin to occur prior to the onset of menopause, during, or after. They include hot flashes, night sweats, irritability, and stress; they can last for months or years. These disturbing symptoms do not make it easy to sleep. They are not only uncomfortable but also stimulate cortisol, which as we know is the "hyperarousal" hormone. Therefore, sleep disturbances are common during this time in a woman's life.

Hot flashes are the result of a surge of adrenalin production in the body, which awakens the brain and causes a rise in body temperature and sweating. Mood swings and depression are also common symptoms that accompany menopause, all of which can lead to insomnia. About 20 percent of women experience depression during menopause. However, there may be other causes for depression, which can further exacerbate menopausal symptoms.[52]

Research has shown that sleep disturbances during midlife are associated with hot flashes, night sweats, and chronic stress. Results on polysonography show that arousal occurs prior to the onset of hot flashes. Other causes of sleep disturbances in middle-aged women are obesity, disordered breathing, and co-morbidities (existing physical or mental conditions). In addition to these common symptoms, there may be other underlying physiological or psychological causes of insomnia at this time of women's life cycle that should be evaluated. Treatment should be targeted to treating the underlying problems and symptoms to improve sleep quality.[53]

Any type of stress, whether it be acute or chronic, is likely to cause insomnia symptoms. It is so easy to talk about "stress," a nebulous term. We all have stress in our lives. The question remains: does stress cause insomnia or does insomnia cause stress? I certainly believe it is both. Disturbances in our bodies, in our lives, and our environment (stressful events or stressors) cause a response in our bodies that triggers a stress response—arousal, alerting, increased heart and respiratory rates, increased blood pressure, and other physical and emotional responses. This stress response works against the calming hormones that promote sleep.

Both the stressor and body response vary in intensity depending on the particular event or pathology. Naturally, if we are aroused, our sleep (or lack of it) is disturbed. If I have the least little worry, I either can't fall asleep or if I do so quickly, I frequently wake up later and then can't fall back to sleep thinking about the things that are bothering me.

Recommended management for menopausal symptoms include good sleep hygiene, such as keeping the bedroom dark and cool and avoiding alcohol, caffeine, tobacco. Also, hormone replacement therapy (HRT) is effective for many women. There is controversy regarding health risks, such as cancer. HRT does relieve many of the disturbing menopausal symptoms and also helps prevent osteoporosis. Sufferers should receive medical attention and education regarding the pros and cons of taking HRTs.

Now that we've concentrated on women's sleep issues through their menstrual cycles, reproductive years, and menopause, here is a word about men. Men of all ages also have sleep problems, just not as frequently as women. Male hormones also play a role. Physical and psychological health problems are major factors in men, as well as women, as causes of sleep disturbances. Underlying causes and parasomnias discussed in chapters 5 and 7, as well as idiopathic insomnia, affect men as well as women. As a matter of fact, obstructive sleep apnea is more prevalent in men than in women (as we will see in the next chapter).

Several research study results have shown that more adult men have greater decreases in slow-wave (deep) sleep than women have. This is paralleled by a decline in growth hormone (GH) secretion. Major growth ceases, following adolescence. In a study published in the *Journal of the American Medical Association* in 2000, investigators sought to determine age-related changes in sleep quality, duration, GH levels, and cortisol levels in 149 healthy men, who had no sleep complaints (aged 16 to 83 years). The results showed that time spent in deep, slow-wave sleep decreased from 19 percent in the 16- to 25-year-old age group to 3.4 percent in the 36- to 50-year-old age group. There was also a marked decrease in the secretion of growth hormone in the midlife to the late-life age group. It is well known that there is a decrease in GH as people age—their growth in height has long stopped. What is also known is that cortisol (the awake hormone) also increases with age and higher amounts are secreted with even partial sleep deprivation.[54]

We have established that sleep disturbances become more prevalent with age. There are various intrinsic (hormones and diseases) and extrinsic (environment and stress) factors that influence sleep as we age. According to Dr. David Neubauer, "Life events, schedule demands, habits and routines, circadian timing predisposition, biological changes, the risk of various disorders (psychiatric, medical, and sleep), medications and substance use all generally may have different influences at different life stages. The end result is the epidemiological evidence showing that the complaint of insomnia increases steadily with age."[55]

Older Adults

Normal aging is associated with changes in sleep quantity, quality, and sleep architecture, such as a decrease in the ability to initiate and maintain sleep and a decrease in the proportion of deep, slow-wave and restorative sleep. These changes may be related to neurocognitive dysfunction, age-related

changes in circadian rhythm, and also changes in homeostatic, cardiopulmo-
nary, and endocrine functions.[56]

Throughout the life cycle there are so many variables—intrinsic physical
changes, health issues, and environmental factors—that affect sleep, so that
all changes in sleep parameters can't be generalized to specific ages. It is
obvious that as people age, they generally have more physiologic changes
occurring in their bodies. Psychological factors, such as loss and grief, also
play a role. In other words we are all deteriorating slowly as we age. (Allen's
tennis is improving at 81, so he says he might want to object to this sentence.)

Sleep disturbances are more common in the elderly than any other life
stage. According to a 2003 National Sleep Foundation survey, 44 percent of
older persons experience one or more symptoms of insomnia at least a few
nights a week or more often. These symptoms include daytime sleepiness,
irritability, depression, and difficulty concentrating. Many elderly adults
report being less satisfied with sleep and feeling more tired during the day.
Research conducted on the sleep habits of older adults show increase in the
time it takes to fall asleep (referred to as sleep latency), decline in the length
of REM sleep, and an increase in sleep fragmentation (times in the night they
wake up).[57]

The most profound change in sleep architecture as people age is the
time spent in deep, slow-wave delta sleep. Whereas 20-year-olds spend about
45 minutes in delta sleep during the first few hours of sleep, by age 60, time
spent in delta drops to only a few minutes each night. More time is spent in
stages 1 and 2. In general, total sleep time only slightly diminishes. Older
adults also wake up more during the night and many have trouble falling back
to sleep. Older people feel that they don't get enough sleep, but it is usually
the quality of sleep that is diminished.[58]

There are so many factors that affect sleep at any age; however, these
are multiplied as people age. The older people get, the more health problems
they encounter, particularly aches and pains related to all sorts of problems.
Pain caused by osteoarthritis, for example, affects so many elders. Our urinary
bladders lose tone, so we have to get up out of warm and cozy beds more frequently to empty our bladders. Biological and physical changes, depression
and a wide variety of physical and mental ailments affect sleep quality as
we age. I generally wake up twice a night to empty my bladder. Sometimes
I fall right back to sleep. Other times I start worrying about falling back to
sleep; then I can't. That is because my "alert" hormones kick in.

According to Neubauer, "Surveys of community-living elders typically
show that more than half report difficulty initiating or maintaining sleep or
persistent early morning awakening." Lab polysomnographic test results have

concurred with these complaints, showing increased arousals. Such evaluations have also confirmed the decrease in time spent in slow-wave (deep) sleep in healthy elders.[59]

The results from a 2003 National Sleep Foundation poll of 1,506 Americans between the ages of 55 and 84 showed that the healthier people of this age group were, the better they slept. Of course, the more health problems people had, the more likely they were to have sleep disorders. Sixty-seven percent of those surveyed in this study reported "having sleep problems at least a few times a week, including difficulty falling asleep, frequent awakenings throughout the night, inability to go back to sleep after an unwanted awakening, pauses in breathing, and unpleasant feelings in their legs."[60]

As seen above, more women than men report symptoms of insomnia from the onset of puberty, through midlife, and into old age. Older men also experience more sleep problems than they did when they were younger. However, their symptoms are more likely due to sleep-related breathing problems and some parasomnias (described in subsequent chapters).

Due to the poor amount of sleep and poor quality of sleep during the night, older people tend to take naps during the day. Daytime napping can lead to negative effects on the body's homeostatic balance and circadian rhythm differentiation between day and night. What happens is that routine napping during the day can distribute sleep intermittently throughout the day and night (similar to newborn babies' patterns). Also, elders lose some of their sleepiness drive in the evening, so there is lack of reinforcement of the circadian differentiation between day and night. Other factors related to changes in elder persons' sleep habits are life changes that occur more frequently as people age. These might be loss of a spouse, other family member, or dear friend; moving to a new residence; or other life change. Another element is a shift in circadian rhythm phase to an earlier time, meaning as people age, they have an earlier morning awakening time. People who have been "morning people" for much of their lives experience this shift more than "night people." This shift occurs to some extent in most elderly people no matter what their previous bio-rhythms have been.[61]

Older people deal with their sleep problems in different ways as revealed from our surveys, described in Chapter 6. Of course, for older people who are retired on adequate incomes, adjustments to these changes in sleep patterns are often not difficult, and sometimes are desirable based on their recreational or creative activity schedules. Certainly, if they are a problem, underlying health problems and sleep disorders should be first evaluated and treated. Sleep medications work for some people, but many choose not to take such medications, sometimes because they are advised by their doctors or the drug information that the sleep medications would interfere with, or act adversely with, other medications that have been prescribed. It is also important to keep in mind that elderly people metabolize medications differently than younger people. Certain medications—including over-the-counter, non-prescription medications—can have adverse effects on people who have health problems that affect the kidney and liver. More about medications and other treatments for insomnia is discussed in Chapter 9.

CHAPTER 5

Sleep Disorders and Underlying Pathologies

Do you have difficulty waking up in the morning and feel unrefreshed and drowsy? Do you tend to doze off while listening to someone talking to you, while watching TV, or even when driving? Do you take repeated naps during the day? Do you feel exhausted, irritable, or depressed? These are all signs of sleep deprivation. You obviously aren't getting enough sleep or the quality of your sleep is very poor. You might be suffering from an underlying disorder that is disrupting the quality and quantity of sleep you should be getting each night. This chapter will cover the known causes of insomnia and poor sleep quality.

As stated earlier, probably several times, insomnia is a symptom of some other problem—most of the time. When there is no underlying problem or specific sleep disorder, then the insomnia is a disorder in itself and is referred to as "primary" insomnia. Symptoms are subjective; that is, they are what the patient feels and explains to the care provider. Sometimes the underlying problem is difficult to establish. Dr. Dement, in his book, *The Promise of Sleep*, declared that "there are so many different types of insomnia, attributable to so many different causes," it is difficult to determine the best treatment; and furthermore, there are too few good scientific studies to determine the best course of treatment.[1]

Transient insomnia—lasting a few days to a week or two—is generally due to worry or anxiety about something that is disturbing, such as family or work-related issues. Worry and stress place the individual in a hyperarousal state. Upcoming happy events can also elicit the arousal state that causes sleeplessness. Other causes might be jet lag, sleeping away from home, and a brief illness. Time zone and work schedule changes disrupt the circadian rhythms, which are thrown out of synchrony.

Chronic insomnia—long-term insomnia that lasts weeks, months, or years—can result from unresolved causes of short-term insomnia. Pain, discomfort of any nature (such as chronic headaches), or any medical problem, such as heart or lung diseases, neurological diseases, diabetes, gastrointestinal reflux, and other diseases, all can disrupt sleep.

Frequent urination, medically referred to as "nocturia," can certainly disturb sleep. People with diabetes, bladder and kidney disorders, or simply "getting older" often need to get up several times during the night to urinate. This obviously disturbs sleep. Some people are fortunately able to get back to sleep, but others aren't always able to do so. I have to get up several times a night and most of the time am able to fall back to sleep. If I start fretting about something, then I am unable to readily fall back to sleep. Whatever the cause, the problem needs to be investigated. If there is a known underlying health problem, it should be treated.

Dr. Dement believes that people who have insomnia every night, without exception, for months or years are very rare. In most cases, insomniacs have problems sleeping for a few nights; then they sleep well some nights, and their problems return again.[2] As stated previously, there are two basic categories of insomnia—primary and secondary insomnias.

Primary insomnia is chronic insomnia without a known underlying cause. There are two categories of primary insomnia—"psychophysiological" and "idiopathic" insomnia.

Psychophysiological insomnia refers to learned or conditioned insomnia. In this case, the individual feels a great deal of tension when getting ready for bed. The tension derives from being unable to sleep on previous nights, anticipating the pattern will continue. This, I know, is basically my problem and most likely many others. *Idiopathic insomnia* (same as primary insomnia) is a lifelong inability to obtain adequate sleep. It is believed to be due to abnormal brain mechanisms that control the sleep-wake cycle.[3] Idiopathic insomnia is also known as true insomnia. It usually begins in childhood and is seen in siblings and parents. Therefore, there may be a genetic connection. Individuals are treated with medication such as low-dose antidepressants and hypnotic medications (sleeping pills).[4] Without a known cause, treatment is geared to alleviating the symptom. Good sleep hygiene should also be adhered to.

Good sleep hygiene means adapting habits that are conducive to sleep, such as maintaining a calm, quiet, and relaxing environment at a chosen bedtime. It is important to go to bed the same time each night and follow a ritual that works best for you in preparing for sleep. Make your room dark and a little cool. Maintain regular bedtime and awake time hours, avoid caffeine after lunch, avoid alcohol beverages near bedtime, and avoid daytime naps.

Poor sleep hygiene refers to people's habits that prevent sufficient sleep and could lead to sleep deficit. Such habits include environment not conducive to sleep, such as too much light or noise, napping during the day, consuming too much caffeine during the day, or drinking an alcoholic beverage in the evening too close to your desired bedtime.

Secondary insomnias are those having an underlying cause that can be diagnosed. These kinds of insomnia generally can be treated once the underlying cause or pathology is established. Here follows specific physiologic and psychosocial disorders that lead to insomnia. In these situations, insomnia is the major symptom.

Delayed sleep-phase syndrome (DSPS) or Advanced sleep-phase syndrome (ASPS), believed to be disorders of the body's biological clock, are out of phase with more natural sleep/awake cycles. People suffering from DSPS have a great deal of difficulty falling asleep in the evening and waking up in the morning. They have sleep-onset insomnia and may not be able to fall asleep until early morning hours and then are unable to wake up early. This is a real problem for people who have to be on their jobs early or attend school or college classes.

DSPS is a chronic disorder of the timing of sleep and body rhythms, such as hormonal processes, core body temperature, and other homeostatic rhythms. Basically, sufferers cannot sleep when sleep is desired, needed, or expected. If they have to get up early because of work or school schedules, they suffer from extreme sleepiness during the day. The prevalence is about 0.15 percent of men and women, but may be as high as 7 percent in adolescents.[5]

Another name for delayed or advanced sleep disorders is "circadian rhythm sleep disorders." Normal circadian rhythms are slightly longer than 24 hours. People who have delayed or advanced sleep-phase disorders seem to have a misalignment of their internal clocks, which run slower or faster than the norm. ASPS is more common in the elderly; the sleep period is displaced to an earlier time. The cause of these disorders is unknown, but one possibility is the sufferers' inability to respond to environmental time cues of darkness and light. People who are blind or work night or swing shifts are more prone to develop these disorders.[6] Some people may secrete a diminished amount of melatonin.

DSPS is common among college students, and sometimes among young children who are in the habit of going to bed late. Such individuals become conditioned to this routine and then are not sleepy if they attempt to go to bed earlier. Their biological clock is alerting, when they finally get ready to go to sleep. These people find it difficult to wake up and feel tired or exhausted during the day. The cause of this disorder is not known, but it does tend to run in families. Some people who have DSPS adapt well if they don't have to get up early. They are alert and are most creative working until the wee hours of the morning.[7] My son and husband are examples of this phenomenon.

It seems that so-called "night people" have DSPS. When my son attended college, he liked to stay up late studying until the wee hours of the morning. He had told me (back then in the 1980s) that it was quiet with the rest of the family asleep. No one disturbed him. He was able to arrange his class schedule so that his first class was at noon. This worked for him and he seemed to get enough sleep. His son, David, whom I've mentioned in Chapter 4, also keeps very late hours. My other grandson, Michael (David's brother), who is 12 years old, also goes to bed late, so it seems to me. There could very well be a genetic connection here. My husband Allen also has strange (in my view) sleep habits, as described in Chapter 3. However, he is really the step-grandfather of David and Michael, so there can be no genetic connection from that side.

It is difficult to diagnose DSPS. Other medical, psychosocial, or psychiatric disorders should first be ruled out. Sleep diaries or logs are useful tools in diagnosing circadian rhythm disorders. A specific questionnaire (MEQ) and polysomnography are used for further diagnosis or to rule out other sleep disorders.

These disorders can be treated by manipulating environmental light and darkness in the bedroom. For DSPS sufferers, exposure to bright light in the early morning and darkness at desired sleep times in the evening have shown to be effective, whereas bright light in the early evening may be effective in delaying sleep in ASPS. Melatonin taken a few hours prior to their desired sleep time effectively advances the time of sleep onset in DSPS.[8]

Restless Legs Syndrome (RLS) is a condition in which the affected individual feels unusual and disturbing sensations in his or her limbs, particularly the legs. These sensations have been described as creeping, crawling, prickly, tugging, tingling, itching, searing, boring, or even painful feelings in their legs. Sufferers of this disorder feel the need to move their legs or get up and move around to obtain relief from the annoying sensations. Because of these disturbing sensations, it is very difficult for them to lie still, to fall asleep or to return to sleep after they have awakened. It is estimated that 5 percent of the U.S. population—an estimated 10 million people—suffer from this problem. It can be devastating. It is the second major sleep disorder after narcolepsy.[9]

Dr. Carlos Schenck, in his book, *Sleep*, contends that RLS is the third most commonly reported sleep disorder, affecting 10 to 15 percent of the population. It is often undiagnosed or misdiagnosed. He stated it "has got to be the biggest completely unaddressed health care priority in America."[10] People suffering from this problem feel they need to move their legs, stretch, or walk to alleviate the disturbing sensations. According to Schenck, "RLS can be maddening, exquisitely painful, and seriously disrupting to sleep quality and duration."[11]

In her book, *Insomniac*, Gayle Greene claimed that RLS can have cataclysmic effects on people's lives. Symptoms sometimes begin in childhood. A definite cause is unknown. However, it is believed to be due to iron deficiency.[12] In July 2007, researchers at the Mayo Clinic found a mutated gene linked to this disorder. The head investigator in this study, Carlos Vilarino-Guell, contended that not all the subjects in the study who had a defective gene had symptoms of RLS. It is possible that there are other triggers for this disorder to be expressed. Dr. Vilarino-Guell stated, "This gene is probably not the most common cause of RLS in the population we studied...."[13]

RLS does seem to cluster in families. A recent Canadian study, conducted at the University of Montreal Hospital Research Center, revealed that sons and daughters of people with RLS were at nearly double the risk of developing this syndrome. The risk to brothers and sisters was nearly fourfold. The researchers determined that family members of a person with RLS have a 77 percent risk of developing the syndrome.[14]

Women are at higher risk than men for having RLS. The problem is also exacerbated by pregnancy. Iron-deficiency anemia is more common in women, and even more so in pregnant women. So it is plausible that more women than men are troubled by RLS. Researchers also find there is an imbalance of dopamine (a brain chemical) in sufferers of RLS. The lead researcher in the Canadian study, Dr. Guy Rouleau, contended that, although this syndrome was first described in the 1950s, "it is the most common disease your doctor doesn't know about."[15]

There are two types of RLS. One is primary (also referred to as idiopathic), in which the cause is unknown or it is familial (inherited). The other type is labeled secondary, meaning there is an underlying cause, such as iron-deficiency anemia (as previously determined) peripheral neuropathy (pathology involving nerves in the legs), an underlying medical condition, or certain medications that can trigger symptoms of RLS.[16] Iron is necessary for the synthesis of dopamine, which was also found to be deficient in the brain. So, this connection is understandable.

Some of the medical conditions known to be able to trigger RLS include chronic kidney failure, peripheral neuropathy, Parkinson's disease, diabetes, and Lyme disease. Medications, such as cold, allergy, and anti-nausea preparations, antidepressants, and anti-seizure and anti-psychotic medications can trigger RLS. Caffeine and nicotine can trigger RLS or aggravate existing symptoms.[17]

RLS can be tormenting to the elderly, particularly if they are confined to chairs, unable to ambulate on their own. Elderly people are more prone to have iron-deficiency anemia because of changes in gastrointestinal functioning, poor nutrition, or loss of appetite.

The first line of treatment is good sleep hygiene. Massaging the affected legs and taking warm baths at bedtime are recommended. Individuals who are troubled by this condition should have a laboratory blood test to determine if they have an iron deficiency. If diagnosed with iron deficiency, they should treated with iron supplements. Underlying medical conditions should, of course, be treated. Other therapies include drugs that stimulate the creation of dopamine in the brain, muscle relaxants, some anticonvulsants, opiates (to relieve pain and other sensations), and some anti-anxiety drugs.[18]

Periodic Limb Movements in Sleep (PLMs) is another sleep disorder related to RLS. It is characterized by brief muscle twitches and/or jerking movements of the feet, ankles, and legs. These movements cluster in episodes lasting from a few minutes to several hours. The cause of this syndrome is unknown, but it is not considered medically serious. It can contribute to chronic insomnia and disturb the sleeping partner. There is no specific treatment, unless accompanied by RLS.[19] About 80 to 90 percent of people who have this problem also have RLS. Episodes generally last about five seconds and recur about every 15 to 40 seconds. Most people aren't aware of their symptoms.[20]

Obstructive Sleep Apnea (OSA) is a serious disorder that affects the quantity and quality of sleep. It is a condition in which muscles in the walls of the pharynx (back of the throat) relax, which causes the upper airway to narrow or become completely occluded, to the extent that the sufferer stops breathing for at least 10 seconds. The term "apnea" actually means cessation of breathing. When this happens, oxygen is not delivered to the brain or other body parts. The brain responds to the oxygen deficit by triggering arousal, forcing the person to wake up briefly. The individual doesn't even remember waking up. This can happen hundreds of times per night, leading to chronic sleep deprivation and daytime sleepiness and exhaustion.[21]

There are two types of sleep apnea. The other less common type is central apnea, which means the brief absence of breathing is due to failure of the brain to send signals to the muscles that control breathing. This type of sleep apnea may occur in pre-term babies who are sent home with monitors. Central sleep apnea also may result from congestive heart failure or high doses of narcotics. The major cause of sleep apnea is obstruction in the airway, because the muscles in the back of the throat fail to keep the airway open sufficiently during inspiration.

Obstructive sleep apnea (OSA) is a potentially life-threatening condition that can cause poor health, such as high blood pressure, cardiovascular disease, and a slew of other medical and mental conditions. More than 18 million Americans are believed to suffer from sleep apnea.[22]

A recent estimate of the prevalence of this condition is that one in five U.S. adults has mild apnea. About one in 15 sufferers has moderate to severe OSA. The risk of developing OSA increases two- to four-fold if there is a family history of this condition. In one study of 1,090 U.S. adults, the researchers concluded that more that 80 percent of men and 90 percent of women with moderate to severe sleep apnea go undiagnosed. It is only in recent years that this disorder is being recognized and addressed by the medical community. More women may have OSA than reported because their symptoms of fatigue and irritability are more likely to be attributed to other conditions, such as depression, hypothyroidism, fibromyalgia, and migraine.[23]

The incidence of OSA increases in women following menopause. The overall incidence also rises as people get older because the muscle walls surrounding the airway decrease in tone. Even more problems trouble the elderly. The oxygen deficit due to the apnea can cause confusion, forgetfulness, cognitive deficits, excessive daytime sleepiness, high blood pressure, and other medical problems. Symptoms in the elderly can easily be misdiagnosed; they are often attributed to Alzheimer's or to depression.[24]

The major symptoms are snoring, gasping, and periods of apnea (no breathing) for at least 10 seconds, throughout the night. The person wakes up due to oxygen deficit, then gasps and breathes, and promptly returns to sleep. The person doesn't realize this is happening, but suffers from major sleep deficit. He or she might suffer from extreme sleepiness during the day, irritability, memory loss, impaired concentration, sexual dysfunction, and depression. In addition, the sufferer frequently has co-morbidities—that is the existence of medical conditions, such as high blood pressure, cardiovascular diseases, and diabetes. The sufferer may not be aware of his loud, tortuous snoring and many periods of apnea, but his (or her) partner surely is aware of it. If the individual lives alone, the problem is not so easily diagnosed.

A recent report from HealthDay News cited a new study linking OSA to higher risks for heart failure and heart disease in middle-aged and older men, but did not find a correlation between OSA and heart disease in women or in men over 70 years old. The study did show that men between the ages of 40 and 70 who had severe apnea were 68 percent more likely to develop heart disease and 58 percent more likely to develop heart failure than those without the condition.[25]

The typical profile of the person who has OSA is a middle-aged, obese male who complains of excessive daytime sleepiness. This cardinal symptom, or an injury sustained at work or while driving, or a request from his partner, are among the reasons that he seeks medical attention.

Sleep-breathing disorders can occur at any age. In young children, partial or total airway obstruction is usually due to enlarged tonsils and adenoids and can also be due to stuffy nose or deviated septum or "other lumps or bumps."[26] Removal of tonsils and adenoids usually fixes the problem.

OSA is one of the most serious general health problems in America. According to Dr. Dement, "Apnea is an unrecognized killer, but it is hiding in plain sight. Every night more than 50 million Americans stop breathing."[27] When breathing stops, less oxygen enters the lungs and the rest of the body. Oxygen deficits in the brain and heart are particularly dangerous. The heart can stop beating; if it stops for 20 seconds or more, it has trouble resuming its beat again.[28] In addition to the risk of severe medical conditions, daytime sleepiness can lead to motor, workplace, and other accidents. It is just about impossible for people with this disorder to make up the enormous sleep deficit without treatment.

Air pollution may be tied to breathing problems during sleep. A recent study was conducted by the Harvard School of Public Health and Brigham & Women's Hospital to investigate if there was a link between air pollution and sleep-disordered breathing. After analyzing the data on 3,000 people, the researchers found that the incidence of sleep apnea and low levels of oxygen during sleep increased as environmental temperature rose and air pollution worsened. The authors concluded that particles of pollution could have negative effects on the central nervous system as well as the upper airways.[29]

The most prominent symptoms of OSA, chronic snoring and complaints of severe exhaustion, generally motivate the individual to seek medical attention. These symptoms alone are not by themselves diagnostic of the condition. Moreover, the sufferer is generally not aware that he or she snores or stops breathing while sleeping. Diagnosis of obstructive sleep apnea can be confirmed in a sleep laboratory in which a series of tests are performed. The group of laboratory tests is referred to as polysomnography. The individual tests include electroencephalography (ECG), electro-oculography (EOG, measurements of eye movements), chin and limb electromyography (measurements of limb movements), respiratory air flow and effort, body position, and oxygen blood saturation. Also, sleep latency, number of awakenings, periods of uninterrupted sleep, and total sleep time are determined.[30]

There are several treatment options for OSA. The main goals of treatment are to improve the pathology and to eliminate or minimize the symptoms. Mild OSA can be managed by some lifestyle changes. Since obesity is a major factor, weight loss is an initial goal. Other behaviors include changing sleep positions, such as sleeping on one's side (instead of back), eliminating alcoholic beverages in the evening, limiting caffeine beverages to the morning, and quitting smoking. Alcohol causes the muscles of the upper airway to relax. Smoking worsens the swelling of the upper airway. Caffeine has a long biological half-life, so even consuming beverages containing caffeine in the afternoon can have a negative effect on sleep.

The treatment of choice is continuous positive airway pressure (CPAP). The apparatus used for this treatment is a bedside device with a blower providing increased air pressure, a tube, and a plastic mask that covers the nose and/or mouth. The air gently flows from the container, through the tube to the mask and into the airway. The gentle pressure of the air flowing into the airway keeps the airway open. Many CPAP machines incorporate humidifiers. Variations include bilevel positive airway pressure (BiPAP) and auto-titrating devices. This method of treatment does take practice and getting accustomed to.

Common complaints from people who use this equipment include discomfort from wearing the mask, nasal dryness, nasal congestion, sinusitis, and stomach discomfort. Improved designs of this equipment and warming the attached humidifier has minimized some of these adverse effects.[31] Compliance is certainly necessary for this treatment to be effective.

Another method of treatment is the use of an oral appliance—a plastic device that fits over the teeth to keep the jaw and tongue forward, elevating the soft palate.[32]

A more drastic treatment option is surgery. There are several surgical procedures that can be performed, depending on the defect in the individual's upper airway. To determine this, an endoscopic examination of the upper airway is performed.

One surgical procedure is uvulopalatopharyngoplasty (UPPP), the medical terminology for surgical removal of the uvula (that little piece of tissue that hangs at the back of the throat), and removing some excess tissue of the pharynx (throat), tonsils, and parts of the soft palate (soft tissue on the rear roof of the mouth).[33]

Other surgical procedures include nasal reconstruction to improve nasal patency, maxillomandibular (bones of the jaw) expansion, laser-assisted uvulopalatoplasty (reconstruction of the uvula and soft palate), and radio-frequency tissue ablation.[34] The radio-frequency tissue ablation procedure uses energy to shrink excess tissue in the back of the throat. The advantage of this procedure is that it is less invasive, bloodless, and can be performed in an out-patient surgical setting.[35]

Complications of surgical procedures can include bleeding and pain.

Anyone considering any one of these options should be given a thorough explanation — of what the procedure entails, what the risks and possible complications are, how effective these measures are, and any other concerns — from his physician. The individual is then able to make a completely informed decision. Individuals undergoing any of these procedures should continue to have long-term, follow-up care.

Pain is disruptive to sleep, obviously. Pain is a symptom of something gone wrong in the body; the cause can be known or unknown. It is a signal or warning of an injury to some part of the body or a disease process. It is important to seek medical attention when pain occurs. If and when a diagnosis is made, the problem is treated, relief is obtained, then the sleep problem is solved. Unfortunately, there are times when all of the medical tests available do not reveal the cause of pain.

One particular illness that causes generalized pain and stiffness of the muscles and joints is fibromyalgia, which has no known cause. People suffering from this disorder have difficulty falling asleep and staying asleep. In addition to widespread pain and insomnia, other symptoms include numbness or tingling of extremities, chronic daytime fatigue, and mood disturbances. Symptoms may wax and wane in severity and duration.

This disorder affects 2 to 6 percent of people worldwide. Eighty to ninety percent of those affected are women. Not only does the pain from this condition make sleep more difficult, but sleep deprivation exacerbates the symptoms. The causes of fibromyalgia are basically unknown. It does appear to occur in people who have had repeated stress injuries, such as automobile or work-related injuries. This disorder also seems to run in families. Fibromyalgia is considered to be in the family of rheumatoid conditions, but is not a true form of arthritis. Some studies have shown a relationship between fibromyalgia and chronic fatigue syndrome, migraine headaches, lupus, and major depressive disorders.[36]

Unfortunately, there are no specific medications for the treatment of fibromyalgia. Some methods that can relieve the symptoms are exercise, massage, and relaxation techniques. For severe symptoms, pain-relieving medication and sleep aids may be prescribed.[37]

Stress and psychological or psychiatric disorders are another group of underlying disorders that can severely disrupt sleep. Certainly any unresolved stress, psychological or psychiatric disorder can cause transient or chronic insomnia. What is stress? It is the body's response to some event, disease, or situation that stimulates physiological changes in our bodies. The events might be "danger" signals in the environment, disturbing personal relationships, work-related situations, or other disturbing events. The trigger (also called the "stressor") can be a disturbing event, a frightening event, or even a happy event.

Our bodies respond to these triggers by eliciting a stress response. "Stress" hormones are released from our brains and adrenal glands (located above our kidneys). Initially, adrenalin and norepinephrine are released, causing our heart rate and blood pressure to rise, our breathing to accelerate, and our pupils to dilate. This is the immediate stress response that prepares us for "fight or flight." It is the survival mechanism that enabled our cavemen ancestors to run away or fight in the face of danger. Once the immediate threat is passed, other hormones are released that allow us to calm down. However, when the stressor persists for extended periods of time, another hormone secreted by the adrenal glands is cortisol, which keeps us in a state of arousal. This persistent hyperarousal state is the underlying cause of chronic insomnia, as well as other health problems.

I know that when I can't sleep, I feel my heart beating fast and I feel anxious. It becomes a vicious cycle. A good question is, are some people anxious because they can't fall asleep when they want to or anxious as a result of their insomnia?

Sleep disturbances are common among people who are depressed or suffer from psychotic disorders, such as schizophrenia and bipolar disorders, anxiety, panic, and post-traumatic stress disorders. An estimated 12.4 million women and 6.4 men in the United States suffer from depression at some point in their lives. Most depressed people suffer from insomnia.[38]

Insomnia is one of the diagnostic symptoms in depression. Sleeplessness, in turn, contributes to depressive disorders. People with depression have a range of insomnia symptoms, which are an inability to fall asleep, an inability to stay asleep, unrefreshing sleep, and daytime sleepiness. Because many times symptoms of insomnia and depression overlap, diagnosis of any one of these disorders is difficult. When individuals are evaluated for symptoms of insomnia, they should also be evaluated for depression. Treatments should focus on both depression and insomnia. Such treatments include both hypnotic and anti-depressant medications.[39]

A 2005 "Sleep in America" poll of the National Sleep Foundation (NSF) found that 18 percent of adults in the 18 to 64 age range who were depressed also had symptoms of a sleep disorder. In the age range, the NSF 2006 poll found that, among those in the age range 11 to 17 who reported feeling unhappy, 73 percent reported that they were not getting enough sleep at night.[40]

As stated several times, insomnia is a symptom of some underlying cause most of the time. However, insomnia can be also idiosyncratic, meaning there is no underlying cause that can be identified (so that it is referred to as primary insomnia, as defined earlier). It is important to be evaluated by your primary health care provider for any underlying conditions or sleep disorders that might cause your insomnia. Basically the management for most insomnias is to first diagnose and then treat the underlying cause, if at all possible. Some sleep experts contend that many providers neglect the evaluation of people's sleep habits and underestimate the importance of sleep for overall health. Good sleep hygiene, as discussed previously, is the first order of beating insomnia. Sometimes medication is indicated. Further management of insomnia and other sleep disorders will be discussed in Chapter 9. The next chapter will deal with individual sleep problems and how these people have managed their insomnia.

CHAPTER 6

Selected Stories from Surveys and Interviews

NOTE TO THE READER: The actual questionnaires, as filled out by the volunteers in our survey, are not included in this book, for privacy reasons discussed in the appendix. A narrative has been written from each questionnaire, the name of the person has been changed for privacy, and each narrative has been numbered, italicized, and placed into the six sleep categories that will be described below before the narratives are presented. Most of the discussion in this chapter about the information in the narratives is printed in ordinary font.

It is not intended that the reader read in sequence all of the narratives in the first reading. Most readers should just read the paragraphs before the narratives, browse through the narratives, particularly those in the same sex and sleep category of the reader, and then read the rest of the chapter and the book. After the narratives, some ways are suggested in this chapter for you to return to the book and read samples of the numbered narratives that might be applicable to your own situation. If it provides any help to compare your situation to those in narratives in other sleep categories, then you may also read additional narratives to find out how others have dealt with or avoided significant sleep problems.

In addition to including a sufficient number of narratives in the book that might help individual readers in various situations, another purpose of including all of these narratives is the possibility that other scientists or physicians might find them of interest for comparison with their own research results.

The purposes of the questionnaires and narratives are described further in Appendix A. This sample of stories was not necessarily expected to provide a "representative" sample, nor any subsample of the American public. Nor was it expected to test any findings of the much larger studies conducted by well-funded research centers. In fact, publications from these authoritative research centers are important sources from which much of the information in this book has been obtained for the reader. However, we believe that you will likely find, qualitatively, that the narratives in this book contain all of the symptoms and effects of insomnia, or of good sleep habits, that you and those among your family and friends might have experienced.

Our population sample is, in fact, skewed toward certain cultural and age ranges. Neubauer indicates that the general cultural expectation of sleep in the Unites States is eight hours during the night.[1] Our convenience sample is taken mainly from in and around the Worcester County area near Ocean City, Maryland, where we live at Ocean Pines. This area is heavily weighted with persons native to the area, those who have settled here in retirement to be near a beach location with its recreational advantages, and students from nearby colleges. One of our best friends who grew up mostly in this area, who has friends and relatives here from her early days in this area, and who returned here about 16 years ago, has described this culture and its effects on sleep patterns as follows:

> In this area it is difficult to identify sleep issues. There is no routine or schedule to develop habits or patterns. Some seasons you work 14 to 18 hours a day, come home, and drop into a sleep of exhaustion. Some seasons we go into hibernation mode where one might say, "I have no trouble sleeping. I slept all day yesterday." Our sleep patterns are also very weather dependent because of farming, fishing, and the construction industry.

This friend's statement refers, of course, to persons native or otherwise, who are working-class families and are affected by available work and work conditions at the resort locations in the area. Different conditions would also apply to the retirees in our sample, who form into different social and/or church groups for a joyful and active retirement.

Nevertheless, it will be seen that the symptoms, causes, effects, and treatments described in other chapters of this book are practically all represented in these narratives from the limited numbers of participants that the authors have been able to contact. This is true despite the fact that most of the respondents come from the authors' own communities.

In reading these narratives, readers might well be helped simply by observing that they are in good company. Sometimes, a reader might occasionally find a useful idea in a context that will help alleviate his own problems with insomnia. If so, the effort to distribute and tell the stories extracted from the questionnaire data has been worthwhile.

Each narrative has been assembled into a few paragraphs that present, in order the basic sleep patterns of the respondent, the causes of these sleep patterns and the effects of sleep loss, and any remedies or medications that have been used, or not used, to change sleep patterns that are unhealthy or disturbing to the respondent. Most of these narratives have, for brevity, been presented in only three paragraphs, in which the causes and effects are given in the second paragraph. The narratives are also grouped according to sex, age, those with no significant sleep problems, those living with sleep problems that might or might not have been found to have some remedies, and those who deem their sleep problems to seriously affect their lives and/or who have sought medical or other professional help. As indicated earlier, names have been changed to fictitious names to ensure privacy.

The reader might also find it interesting to compare experiences with those of others by using the insomnia card game presented at the end of this chapter.

Women's Experiences

Women Who Feel They Have No Sleep Problems

NARRATIVE 23 — CONSTANCE (AB 5/18/10)

Constance was 18 at the time she completed the questionnaire. She has no problem falling asleep but does not get enough sleep about 2 days per week because she is a freshman in college and her course schedule varies from day to day. She goes to bed about midnight or 1 A.M. and, without engaging long in other activities, she falls asleep within 5 or 10 minutes. She now gets up at 8:30 or 11 A.M. depending on her schedule. She never wakes up before arising in the morning.

The causes of her loss of sleep are staying up late and getting up early in the morning. She sometimes talks in her sleep or has nightmares. Sometimes when she is falling asleep she pictures herself walking and then tripping, so she flings forward and wakes herself up. She worries over sleep loss when she does not get enough sleep, but when there are no classes she sometimes can sleep until 2 P.M. Nightmares occur on days when she gets only a couple of hours of sleep. When she does not get enough sleep she feels tired and exhausted until late afternoon or evening.

She takes no medications or treatments to improve sleep.

NARRATIVE 24—ALICE (AB 5/18/10)

Alice was 18 at the time she completed the questionnaire. She indicates that she has no difficulty in falling asleep. She goes to bed around midnight on weekdays and about 3 A.M. on weekends. She might read or engage in other activities in bed for about an hour, and then falls asleep about 20 minutes after turning off the lights. She has no problems with waking during the night and not going back to sleep. She gets up, according to her present schedule in college, at 9:30 A.M. on Mondays, Wednesdays, and Fridays, and at 8:00 A.M. on Tuesdays and Thursdays. However, for months, she has had problems about one night per month. She occasionally will wake up continuously throughout the night without knowing why; usually, she falls back to sleep each time she wakes up, but worries about how many more hours she will be able to sleep.

She believes that the cause of her occasional sleep problem is the stress from having a lot to do the next day, or the stress still felt after a busy day. She has been told that she talks in her sleep all the time, but this does not usually wake her up. Only a few times has she awakened herself by talking in her sleep; these are times when she dreams she is falling. Her occasional nights of insufficient sleep typically do not interfere at all with her day.

Apparently, her occasional sleep problems are not serious. She has no effects from sleep loss and has tried no medications or therapy.

Alice provided an additional narrative to the questionnaire that might be of interpretive interest. It is quoted as it was written:

> *I was asleep in my bed at home when I heard someone rustling around the kitchen. I was completely conscious but couldn't move. I heard it come down the hallway but I couldn't reach over to my cell phone to call my dad who was asleep upstairs. I felt serious pressure over my shoulder and I could not move but I was terrified. Finally I screamed out "Jesus Christ!" and I woke up immediately. My house power had gone out, although the lights in the neighborhood were still on. After a minute our power came on and I calmed down, although I have never had another experience like that!*

Although she indicated in the second sentence that she was conscious, it seems that she must have been in REM sleep, as described in Chapter 2, in which she was paralyzed, although dreaming that she was awake at the time.

NARRATIVE 30—LORENA (AB 5/27/10)

Lorena was 21 when she completed the questionnaire. She does not indicate any difficulty with going to sleep when she goes to bed. She usually goes to bed at 11 P.M., never reads or engages in other activities before turning off the lights, takes only about 10 minutes to go to sleep, and does not have any problem waking up during the night and not going back to sleep. She wants to wake up at 10 A.M., but needs to wake up at 7 A.M. some days to get to class in college.

She does not have sleep problems unless she stays up too late for a reason. She lists no usual causes of sleep loss. Very infrequently she does not get sufficient sleep. On these rare days, she feels very tired, especially in the afternoon about 2 to 3 P.M., and cannot concentrate. However, she often feels tired but it is not related to loss of sleep.

She has taken neither medications nor any other aids for sleeping.

NARRATIVE 32—ESTHER (AB 5/29/10)

Esther was 21 when she completed the questionnaire. She has no difficulties with sleep. She usually goes to bed at 1 A.M. and falls asleep within 10 minutes. She wants or needs to get up at 9 A.M. Sometimes she wakes up at 6 A.M. and is awake for 1 hour. About once or twice a month she does not get quite enough sleep.

On the infrequent times that she has sleep loss, she attributes it to stress over excess work or study, or occasionally to nightmares. She then feels tired the next day with some lack of energy.

She has taken no medications or other remedies because she has no concern over loss of sleep.

NARRATIVE 29—MARILYN (AB 5/26/10)

Marilyn was 42 when she completed the questionnaire. She does not report times of going to bed, times in bed before turning out lights, times to go to sleep or other aspects of her sleep schedules, because she apparently is not concerned about them. The only thing she provides is that every day she wakes up at 2 to 3 A.M. and has trouble going back to sleep.

She cites no causes of her waking during the night, and says, "It just happens." She has been waking up and cannot sleep afterward. However, she is alert during the daytime, and at night she is also alert. She indicates that she does not have a problem sleeping; she states, "I am fine with it." She has no detrimental effects of waking too early. We must assume that she gets enough rest.

Of course, she does not take any medications or remedies to help her sleep.

NARRATIVE 41—MILLIE (AB 8/17/10)

Millie was 44 when she completed the questionnaire. She has excellent sleep habits and no serious difficulties with sleep. In summer when she is not teaching she goes to bed at 11 P.M.; during the school year she is in bed by 10 P.M. She reads or watches comedy before going to bed. She usually reads or engages in other activities in bed for about 30 to 40 minutes before turning off the lights. After turning off the lights, she falls asleep within 15 to 20 minutes. She needs to get up for work at 6 A.M. during the school year, and 8 A.M. in the summer. Occasionally, about once every two weeks, she wakes up at 2 A.M., but falls back to sleep within 30 minutes or less. She seldom wakes up and then has trouble falling back to sleep.

The causes of her infrequent sleep problems are hormonal changes associated with perimenopause, as confirmed by medical tests. Restless leg syndrome can keep her awake, while night sweats will wake her up. These causes of sleep loss occur only two to three days a month. Although she might lose sleep on these infrequent occasions and have trouble waking up the next day, she usually feels alert regardless of the amount of sleep she has had on these occasions.

When she has night sweats, she adjusts the temperature and uses a fan. On occasion when she is too wound up to sleep, she takes Tylenol PM. She states that sleep is an area of life that she does well. She needs to get adequate sleep in order to perform well in teaching. She plans sleep as she does student lessons. She does not drink alcohol, eats well, and is physically very active. She always goes to bed the same time and allows for eight to nine hours of sleep time. She never stays out late, drinks alcohol, or smokes.

This respondent presents the best case of "good sleep hygiene" described so far.

NARRATIVE 4—BUNNY (AB 4/10/10)

Bunny was 63 when she completed the questionnaire. She was unusual in indicating that she never had sleep problems. She goes to bed at 10:30 to 11 P.M., and falls asleep within 5 minutes. She gets up at 7:00 to 8:00 A.M., and does not wake up too early without being able to get back to sleep. Although she does get up occasionally to use the bathroom, she returns to sleep in a short period of time.

NARRATIVE 6—LONNIE (AB 4/12/10)

Lonnie was 64 at the time she filled out the questionnaire. She goes to bed about 10 to 11 P.M. and falls asleep within ten minutes. She gets up to go to the bathroom usually once and usually gets back to sleep within minutes. She gets up at 7 to 8 A.M. She never wakes up too early or has trouble getting back to sleep.

On rare occasions, when she has something on her mind or her joints ache, she loses some sleep and feels somewhat tired the next day, with a lack of energy. Then, she might take a pain/sleep medication.

She usually sleeps pretty well.

NARRATIVE 38—JOLEEN (AB 8/2/10)

Joleen was 70 when she completed the questionnaire. She expresses no difficulties with sleep problems because she always catches up on any sleep loss. She goes to bed between 10:30 and 11:30 P.M., after sometimes watching TV news for one half-hour. She falls asleep right after turning off lights. The times she needs or wants to wake up range between 5 and 8 A.M., depending on the day's work or activities. Occasionally, she wakes up at 3 to 4 A.M., and either thinks about things to do, indulges in creative thinking, reads, or lets her mind just drift through other random issues or images. This early awakening occurs about 10 times a month during her busiest season of activities.

The causes of her occasional early awakening are usually the tasks to be performed during her busy season of activities. If she gets less than 8 hours of sleep on those days, she sometimes begins to tire about 3 P.M. and require a period of relaxation to get her second wind. She indicates that, in any case, she is always able to catch up on any sleep loss, and does not consider that she has any sleep problems.

She takes no medications nor other sleep help, and does not feel she needs any. She seems to have a well-organized life.

Women Who Live with Minor Sleep Problems That Are Well Managed

NARRATIVE 26—EVELYN (AB 5/18/10)

Evelyn was 21 when she completed the questionnaire. Evelyn has sleep problems almost every night. She has had sleep problems for years, since she was in high school. She is a junior in college and also works evenings. Although she might feel tired after work, she usually does not fall asleep for hours. She usually goes to bed about 4 to 5 A.M., after reading or engaging in other activities (studying?) for a couple of hours before turning off the lights. She does not have enough time to go to sleep earlier. Sometimes she will be doing something or watching TV after work and suddenly realize it is 4 A.M. and she must go to sleep. However, sometimes she will go to sleep at 1 to 2 A.M. if she is really tired. After turning off the lights, she falls asleep within

15 to 20 minutes. When she sometimes awakens too early, it is usually about 8 or 9 A.M., and then she does not fall back to sleep but gets up at 10 A.M. She would like to sleep until noon, but needs to get up by 10 A.M. It seems that Evelyn must usually get along on only 4 to 5 hours of sleep in order to continue in college while working nights.

The causes of her loss of sleep seem to be her overload of work and study requirements. She also mentions that sometimes restless leg syndrome keeps her awake. She has been told by friends that she talks in her sleep and carries on conversations. She has also answered the telephone in her sleep and carried on a conversation without remembering any of it. Loss of sleep makes her feel very tired in the mornings and not wanting to get out of bed.

She has not taken any medications or therapies to help herself sleep. Although she usually feels tired in the evenings, she must stay awake at work even though it will sometimes revive her and cause her to stay awake all night. She feels that she does not have enough time during the day to catch up on sleep or does not need to sleep during the day. She also feels that she has more important things to do than sleep. Thus, Evelyn has learned to live with her insomnia.

NARRATIVE 31—KAREN (AB 5/27/10)

Karen was 22 when she completed the questionnaire. Karen indicates that her sleep problems occur only about 4 nights per month, but she has had sleep problems throughout her life, particularly when she is concerned about an obligation or meeting to attend the next day. She wakes up early in anticipation of not missing her obligation, even though she has not had a problem missing any. She usually goes to bed between midnight and 2 A.M.; sometimes her inability to go to sleep makes her delay bedtime. She engages in activities in bed only for about 20 minutes before turning off lights, and then usually falls asleep within 10 minutes. If she needs to get up to go to the bathroom, it takes 15 minutes or so to get back to sleep. She sometimes wakes too early and stays awake from about 5 to 7 A.M.

Her causes of occasional sleep problems are her erratic schedule in college, the fact that she is a light sleeper and easily awakened, nightmares, difficulty clearing her head, and worry over sleep loss. Anxiety about falling asleep often makes her unable to sleep. She thinks some of this might be familial, because her mother is also a late night person and they often stay up together and sleep later in the morning when possible. When she does not get sufficient sleep, she feels cranky and tired, and has difficulty concentrating on matters at hand.

She has taken sleeping pills but they have not worked and leave her feeling groggy the next day. She has also tried to regulate her sleep schedule. However, now that classes are over, she is aware of improvements in her sleep habits.

NARRATIVE 36—LIBBY (AB 7/5/10)

Libby was 41 when she completed the questionnaire. She seems to have had a mild sleep problem for the past two years. For about 12 days a month, her sleep pattern is as follows. She goes to bed about midnight but does not think her bedtime causes her sleep problems. She reads or watches TV in bed for about one hour before turning off the lights. She then tosses and turns for at least an hour before falling asleep. About 3 times a week, she wakes up at 4:30, 5:30, or 6:30 A.M., and then cannot fall back to sleep before arising. She usually needs or wants to wake up by 8 A.M.

The causes of her sleeplessness are related to having too much on her mind. She lists no other physical or mental problems. Her worries are about paying bills in this tough economy, and taking care of her disabled mother who now lives with her. On the days she loses needed sleep, she feels very tired when she first wakes up, then does well the rest of the morning and afternoon until about 3:30 to 4:30 P.M., when she feels like taking a nap.

She takes no medications or self-treatments and has not sought medical help. She thinks going to bed earlier or turning off TV sooner might help.

NARRATIVE 3—DONNA (AB 4/10/10)

Donna was 43 when she completed the questionnaire. The time at which she goes to bed is very variable and depends on her daily schedule of tasks or work, and when she actually feels sleepy. She sleeps best when she allows her body to decide when to sleep. After she goes to bed she does not watch TV or read, because it wakes her and keeps her up. When she goes to bed, she falls asleep within minutes, but she sometimes wakes up early in the morning and cannot go back to sleep. When she wakes up, she stays up. Her sleep problems have been reduced to a couple of times a month in the last five years.

When she occasionally has sleep problems, there can be many causes. Anxiety over some issue affects her sleep. She also occasionally has nightmares, or walks or talks in her sleep. There seems to be no rhyme or reason for occasional sleep problems. She says that when she was a child, she was a "dangerous" sleep walker, actually leaving the house sometimes and requiring better door security. In her teens, she would also walk and eat in her sleep, for which she blames teenage diets. On occasion, she can still walk in her sleep, finding herself awakened in her car, on the couch, in another room, and on one occasion in the hammock. However, she has not been told of any sleep walking/eating episodes in the past two years. Apparently, she might have conquered her parasomnia.

She says that sleeping pills scare her. She is usually very hyperactive but not focused when she does not get enough sleep. However, she takes advantage of short naps when she can.

NARRATIVE 28 — NEENA (AB 5/26/10)

Neena was 63 when she completed the questionnaire. She has sleep problems about 15 times a month. She goes to bed between 12:30 and 3:30 A.M., reads or engages in other activities for variable times, sometimes for two to three hours, and then falls asleep within minutes to hours. After she falls asleep, she usually does not wake up during the night until waking in the morning. She then sleeps until about 7 A.M., always getting up between 7:30 and 9 A.M., not being able to sleep any more in the mornings, even on days she does not need to go to work. This is her main problem. She would like to sleep until 8:30 to 9:30 A.M. She has had these problems for years.

The main causes of her sleep loss are the four nights at work each week. After working, she comes home and needs to unwind before going to bed. During bedtime, she has some arthritic pain, mild restless leg syndrome that she attributes possibly to lack of potassium, and depression that she does not think causes her sleep loss. She usually gets only four to seven hours' sleep on nights she has insomnia, but she still finds herself unable to take naps in the afternoon, except at about 5 P.M. when she feels sleepy but needs to go to work. Her sleep loss is a serious concern and she worries about it. She usually feels tired the day after losing sleep, and cannot get done all the things she wants to do. On the other hand, she sometimes feels great the next day and even seems to have more energy.

Her remedies include rest during the afternoon, but she can never fall asleep; otherwise, she feels that she could make up for her sleep loss. She had taken sleeping pills, such as Tylenol PM, in past years and they worked, but she does not like to take mediations and has not taken them for years. Martinis on the three nights she does not work have helped. Exercise also helps. She seems to live and function, even with insomnia.

NARRATIVE 10 — CARLA (AB 4/13/10)

Carla was 66 when she completed the questionnaire. She very seldom has trouble falling asleep after going to bed at about 10 P.M., but has problems with limited sleep about half of any month. Her sleep problems are unrelated to any activities before she turns off the lights. She tends to arise at 6 A.M. She has problems falling asleep only after a social gathering or when she is overly tired. She will often wake up between midnight and 3 A.M., and sometimes not be able to get back to sleep. She has had sleep problems for about 28 years.

Her sleep problems began when her marriage began falling apart, and were further exacerbated by night sweats during menopause. As menopause approached and other issues occurred, she never was able to sleep through the night; she would be awake when her alarm rang at 4 A.M. When she was working, she would often go to work exhausted and depleted of energy most days, only feeling her potential during rare occasions of good sleep. After retirement, she still had sleep problems, but could better organize her time to recuperate. Causes of sleeplessness include stress, sadness, and other subconscious issues. When losing sleep she still feels exhausted and sometimes very agitated, even in her retirement.

She sometimes uses Excedrin PM to help induce sleep. She has never sought medical assistance because she knows that the issues that interrupt her sleep will always be there. On the other hand, she does not let her sleepless nights affect her upbeat and positive attitude about life. She remains an optimist and surrounds herself with positive relationships and experiences.

NARRATIVE 5—DOLLY (AB 4/12/10)

Dolly was 66 at the time she completed the questionnaire. She goes to bed between 10:30 and 11:30, expecting to get up at 6 or 6:30 A.M. Her night sleep problems occur only 3 or 4 times per month now, but were more frequent until she retired four years ago. If she falls asleep before bedtime then she is wide awake and has difficulty going to sleep. She watches TV or reads for about a half hour before going to bed. Sometimes she gets up to go to the toilet and then cannot go back to sleep, tossing and turning.

The causes of her sleeplessness can be worrying about something she is responsible to do, someone else arising earlier and disturbing the quiet, getting up to go to the bathroom, and sometimes palpitations. Drinking wine at night can sometimes help her go to sleep, but it also later causes wakefulness. Her sleep problems are not severe now that she is retired, but lack of sleep can take off her "edge" and cause a loss of the sense of well-being, a lack of feeling refreshed and rejuvenated.

She does not take sleep medications, but tries reading, thinking, and praying, and usually refraining from wine to help her sleep better.

NARRATIVE 8—ELLEN (AB 4/12/10)

Ellen was 67 when she completed the form. She goes to bed about 8:30 to 9:30 P.M., reads for about 10 to 15 minutes, and then usually falls asleep immediately. She gets up at 6 A.M. During the night, she might awaken at 1:30, 3:30, or 4:30. If she is awakened around 3:30, she is unable to go back to sleep, so she reads until about 5 A.M. Her sleep problems occur only about 5 to 6 times a month.

The causes of her sleep problems include work-related stress or arguments with family or friends. She has also had sleep apnea for the past two years, and has been depressed off and on for a lifetime. When she wakes and is unable to go back to sleep she is annoyed but not frantic. The effects when she loses sleep are tiredness (which she considers a normal state), irritability, and decreased work productivity.

She has not sought medical treatment, but has taken 250 mg of magnesium oxide before bedtime to decrease wakefulness. She has also taken antidepressants. When she wakes with anxiety, aware of a rapid heartbeat and a jittery feeling, she will try reading as a distraction. She usually goes to bed earlier after a previous night of sleep loss.

NARRATIVE 20—RENA (AB 5/13/10)

Rena was 68 when the questionnaire was completed. She goes to bed at 11 P.M., reads or engages in some activity for five minutes and falls asleep within about five minutes. She has no difficulty in falling asleep. She wants or needs to get up at 6 A.M., but about eight times per month she gets up about 4 A.M. to go to the bathroom and is unable to get back to sleep. She is then awake from 3 or 4 A.M. and stays awake for the rest of the day.

She indicates that the causes of her sleep problems are Parkinson's Disease and arthritis. She wakes up with very painful leg cramps that will only stop if she stands up. In addition to pain, she also lists restless leg syndrome, sleep apnea, and depression as causes of her inability to fall asleep again on those nights when she wakes up too early. The days after she loses sleep, she feels tired and sleepy the next day, especially in the late afternoon. The sleep problem was much worse before she retired and needed to work during the day.

In order to improve sleep, she has tried the CPAP machine for apnea, but received little improvement. Getting up and moving around relieves pain, but she is then fatigued the next day; she prefers the fatigue rather than the pain. She does not take pills. Sometimes she stays up late, but it does not help. Swimming and exercise help the most.

NARRATIVE 22—JUNE (AB 5/17/10)

June was 69 when she completed the questionnaire. Often, she sleeps right through the night. She has sleep problems only about seven or eight times per month, either taking longer to fall asleep or waking too early without being able to go back to sleep. She usually falls asleep about 11 P.M. or after, watching TV with a sleep timer turning it off. She occasionally wakes up at 1 A.M., remaining awake for two to three hours, or at about 4 A.M. without going back to sleep. Whatever time she falls asleep, she still awakens about 6 to 6:30 A.M.

She does not know the causes of her sleep problems, which have been occurring for about five years. She has had night sweats and rare instances of restless leg syndrome. She did take Premarin for years, and she seems to feel that this is the reason she has night sweats now. The day after she has lost sleep, she functions but not with vitality. She will feel edgy and in a fog.

She has tried aspirin and sleeping pills such as Tylenol PM, but these medications do not always work. She has found that the best thing to do in the middle of the night if she cannot sleep is to get out of bed and read until she gets tired.

NARRATIVE 27—ETHEL (AB 5/26/10)

Ethel was likely over 70 when she completed the questionnaire; she did not give her age. She does not usually have difficulty falling asleep, except three or four times a month. She goes to bed between 10 and 11 P.M., reads or is active for about one half-hour before turning off lights, and falls asleep within half an hour. She always wakes up between 1 and 3 A.M., is frequently still awake until between 5 and 6 A.M., sometimes falling back to sleep for awhile, but then wanting to get up about 7 A.M.

She lists the cause of her sleep problems as living alone after the death of her husband. After her several sleepless nights a month she feels tired and depressed. She has anxiety and worries over her lost sleep.

Her only remedy is listed as taking one Ativan tablet during the night to return to sleep. The way she deals with her sleep loss several times a month indicates that she likely should be classified as "living with insomnia."

NARRATIVE 12—ELISE (AB 4/14/10)

Elise was 75 years old at the time she completed the questionnaire. She indicated that she has had sleep problems since her thirties, with a frequency of about 7 to 12 nights per month. She goes to bed at 11 P.M. to midnight, and wants or needs to get up at 7 to 8 A.M. Before turning off the lights after going to bed, she occupies herself with reading, prayer, and any other activity only about 15 to 30 minutes. Sometimes, but not all the time, she has difficulty going to sleep; it varies mostly with the moon cycles now, but used to occur on a monthly cycle. The amount of time it takes her to go to sleep after turning off the lights also varies with moon cycles. Her sleep problems are that she occasionally wakes up too early, about 2 to 3 A.M., and is up for 1–3 hours or more. This problem does not occur too often, but usually when she goes to bed too early.

The causes of her occasional sleep problems include the stimulation of watching late night TV or reading late, worrying over what needs to be accomplished the next day (which gets worse the longer she stays awake), and sometimes a feeling of depression. She had thought the problems would diminish after menopause, but now they are related to the moon phases, which can "drive me nuts." After a night of sleep problems, she feels like she has been "dragged through a nuthole and back again." She remains tired and irritable until at least noon.

Her attempts to alleviate the sleep problems, which sometimes help, include behavior modification, avoiding anything disturbing after 9 P.M., breathing exercises and meditation, calming instrumental music, and especially getting enough exercise during the day. They are sometimes effective, and she "lives with" her insomnia.

NARRATIVE 33—DARLENE (AB 5/31/10)

Darlene was 76 when she completed the questionnaire. Darlene has had sleep problems just about every day for many years. She goes to bed between 11:30 and 12:30, watches TV in bed for 15 to 30 minutes, and then takes one or more hours to go to sleep. She usually wakes up between 2 and 4 A.M. and then finds it hard to go back to sleep. She has no special time that she needs to get up in her retirement.

Her main cause of sleep is that her mind keeps working overtime. Other problems with sleep are talking in her sleep, night sweats, nightmares, anxiety, and worry over sleep loss. The detrimental effect of sleep loss is that she feels tired almost every day.

She has taken Tylenol PM to help her sleep, and this has worked sometimes. She has tried a few prescription medications but is limited in what she can take because she takes Coumadin. She does not seem to be suffering greatly in her situation, and seems to be "living with insomnia."

NARRATIVE 16—BERNADETTE (AB 4/17/10)

Bernadette was 85 when she completed the questionnaire. She goes to bed between 10:30 and 11 P.M., and does not read before turning off the lights.

However, she finds it difficult to fall asleep. Without taking a pill she will be awake for three hours; with a pill she might fall asleep within half an hour. She gets up at 6 or 7 A.M., never having slept past 3 A.M., and gets only three to four hours' sleep every night. This has been going on for over five years.

The only causes of sleep loss that she lists are sometimes depression, anxiety, or worry over sleep. She cannot turn off energy or thinking of a specific problem. Although she only gets three to four hours of sleep per night, and she feels some tiredness and mild memory loss (which she attributes possibly to aging), she does not feel tired during the day.

She states that no sleeping pill on the market has been effective in completely improving her sleep habits, although she indicated that a pill reduces her wakefulness from three hours to one hour after turning off lights. She has just decided to live with the problem.

Women Who Have Concerns or Difficulties with Sleep Problems

NARRATIVE 15 — MARIAN (AB 4/15/10)

Marian was 45 when she completed the questionnaire. Her bedtime varies widely but she gets up in the morning between 8 and 9 A.M. She usually reads or engages in other activities for one to two hours before turning off lights, and then it takes 30 minutes to several hours to fall asleep. She often wakes between 3:30 and 4:30 A.M. and cannot go back to sleep. She has sleep loss about 8 to 10 nights per month, a situation that has lasted for about 20 years.

Her causes of sleep loss include apnea, worries over sleep loss, chronic pain, night sweats, nightmares, and depression. She also writes, "It doesn't help when you have a sleep partner who snores." Her nights of sleep loss result in a poor temperament and daytime sleepiness.

She has tried many different prescription and over-the-counter medications, but without much success. Hypnotherapy worked for several years, and she thinks she might try that again.

NARRATIVE 2 — BETH (AB 4/9/10)

Beth was 53 at the time her sleep information was provided. Her main sleep loss occurs only five nights per month, but she has some continuing problems that make her feel tired every day, although she tries to function as necessary. She goes to bed and falls asleep around 10 P.M. during weekdays, but stays up to about midnight on weekends. Sometimes she falls asleep instantly; other times it takes about 10 to 15 minutes. Her bedtime is not related to the sleep problems.

The main cause of her sleep problems is concern about financial problems. This results in some feelings of depression or anxiety. She also has menopausal night sweats. Her only therapy is the use of Advil PM on weekends.

Her biggest concern is that every night she wakes numerous times, looks at the time on the clock, counts how many hours before her alarm will go off (during the week), then rolls over and goes back to sleep. She has never just closed her eyes and slept through the night. She often wakes up at 4:30 or 5:00 and cannot go back to sleep for the rest of the night, arising for work at 6 A.M. on weekdays. She yearns for a full night of sleep.

NARRATIVE 7 — SHERRY (AB 4/13/10)

Sherry was 63 when she answered the questionnaire. She goes to bed about 11 to 11:20 P.M. and has no difficulty going to sleep when she goes to bed, usually falling asleep within five minutes after turning off the lights. She gets up in the morning about 7 to 7:30 A.M. However, she wakes up about 3 to 4 A.M., goes back to sleep in 15 to 30 minutes, and repeats waking and going back to sleep in one- to two-hour intervals until she arises in the morning. She has had sleep problems since she began menopause, but the number of times she is awakened during the night varies.

She attributes her sleep problems to menopause, and the consequent night sweats. She was always a good sleeper until then. The effect of sleep loss is that sometimes she is more tired and less sharp mentally when more wakefulness occurs during the night.

After menopause set in, she slept only about four to five hours total when she would wake up several times during the night. When she was put on hormone replacement therapy (HRT), her sleep problems went away unless there was some unusual stress. When she had her first blood clot, she was removed from HRT and her night sweats and sleep problems returned. She then took over-the-counter (OTC) sleep remedies, such as soy, black cohash, and red clover, but they helped only somewhat. Her gynecologist became concerned about the hormones that were in the OTC remedies, so she was then put back on HRT for six years, and with a lesser dose for six months. With the lesser dose, the sleep problems returned. However, within a month of returning to the original dose, a second blood clot was found, and HRT was stopped. Sleep problems resumed again. Now, she is on an anti-depressant, which helps somewhat, but she still wakes up two to three times a night with hot flashes and night sweats.

NARRATIVE 17—SHANNON (AB 4/17/10)

Shannon was 67 when she completed the questionnaire. She goes to bed between 11 P.M. and 12 A.M., but hates going to bed with the fear that she will have another bad night of insomnia. When she goes to bed the lights are already off; her husband goes to bed at 9 to 9:30 P.M. She is beginning to think that the time she goes to sleep could be a problem; if she stays up later, she finds it harder to go to sleep. How long it takes her to go to sleep also depends on how tired she is. She does not wake up much during the night at present, but she does sometimes get up at 4 A.M. and goes back to bed within the hour. She gets up at 8 or 9 A.M. She has had these sleep problems about half the nights for about 30 years. She takes her problems to bed and creates another problem—no sleep and another bad day. Her husband thinks that her sleep problems are "really rough."

Her sleep problems began when her first husband was having an affair and she was going through a divorce. She was lying in bed without being able to sleep. Her insomnia continued throughout life, including when she was alone for 12 years. Her sleep problems remained even after she remarried and have remained for 23 years of her second marriage.

The causes of her sleep problems include pain sometimes from fibromyalgia, sometimes restless leg syndrome, depression, talking in her sleep, and worrying about sleep. Her husband tells her that she sometimes talks in her sleep. Loss of sleep causes worry, anxiety, fibromyalgia, and more depression.

A big issue was her hearing loss, which began at high frequencies in her twenties and became profound in middle age. She had a cochlear implant four years ago that helps. To treat her insomnia, she has tried psychotherapy, sleep tapes, yoga, exercise, and Ambien. She has been in therapy for depression several times, continues therapy for her sleep issues, and is no longer taking Ambien to help her sleep. She frequently uses Flexeril at night to relieve her fibromyalgia, and feels she is doing better. She is trying to go to bed about the same time each night. She enjoys quiet time at night and watches TV with earphones and closed captioning. She has also been dealing with cancer for the past year but feels she is all right at this time. She has not found a permanent cure for her insomnia, but is doing better now.

NARRATIVE 42—BESS (AB 8/24/10)

Bess was 68 when she completed the questionnaire. She goes to bed at various times, usually between 9 to 11 P.M., but does not think time to bed is related to her sleep problems. She keeps on various night lights when going to bed because she cannot sleep in total darkness at all. After going to bed, she watches TV for an hour or two until she gets sleepy. The time it takes to fall asleep varies, but she usually falls asleep about 10:30 to 11 P.M. Then, she wakes up at about 12 to 12:30 A.M. and the pattern repeats throughout most of the night: sleeping 1 to 1.5 hours, then being awake for 0.5 to 1 hours, then back to sleep, and so on. However, she does seem to sleep better between 5 and 7 A.M., and gets up between 8 and 8:30 A.M. She has had such sleep problems every night for the past 15 years.

The causes she identifies that contribute to her sleep problems are many: difficulty finding a comfortable position; spasms in her feet, legs, and other areas; difficulty with anxiety and "turning off her mind"; pain; nightmares; talking in her sleep; and various medical problems she did not identify. She did not have trouble sleeping soundly when she was young, except that sometimes she walked or talked in her sleep and it wakened her. When her children were young, she seemed to be awakened easily by them during the night. The effects of her sleep loss, which occurs in similar time intervals between successive times of sleep through the night, are that she does not feel mentally or physically alert the next day. Her energy just comes in spurts. She is tired and does not function well in the morning. However, she does well in the afternoon until 5 P.M., and then functions well later in the evening. Her sleep problems have been severe enough that she was forced to retire several years before she would have received her retirement benefits.

Over the years, doctors have given her several prescription drugs. They helped a little, but she has often been allergic to them. She tried melatonin, but that did not help. She has also tried hot baths, drinking warm milk at night, and heat pads for pain, but none of these has relieved the ongoing problems with sleep that still bother her.

Men's Experiences

Men Who Feel They Have No Sleep Problems

NARRATIVE 25—KEVIN (AB 5/18/10)

Kevin was 20 when he completed the questionnaire. Although Kevin indicated no specific times when he went to bed or activities in bed, he seemed to have no problems with his sleep patterns. He could fall asleep within 10 to 30 minutes after going to bed. Sometimes, however, he might wake up at 2:30 A.M. and not go back to sleep. He wants to get up at 10:30 A.M. but sometimes wakes up at 11 A.M., for his scheduled classes as a junior in college. He has a sleep problem only about once a month.

The only cause of some sleep loss that he notes is that he sometimes takes a nap during the day. However, even when losing some sleep, he is fine the next day. He is usually a very alert and energized person. He did relate that when he was about 12 years old, he once dreamed that he was falling off a cliff and woke up to find himself falling out of bed onto the floor. Another time he dreamed that he was talking with his brother and all of a sudden his brother starting making honking noises and he could not understand him; he awoke to find that it was his alarm clock going off.

He has not needed nor taken any sleep medications or therapy.

NARRATIVE 40—RAMSEY (AB 8/17/10)

Ramsey was 46 when he completed the questionnaire. He indicates no difficulty in falling asleep when he goes to bed. He goes to bed between 10 and 11, usually watches TV in bed for 20 to 30 minutes, and then turns off the lights and falls asleep within 10 minutes. He needs to get up for work at 7 A.M. He writes that he is very active physically and has two jobs. He almost always enjoys a good night's sleep, unless he is ill, which is very infrequent.

Ramsey checked off no causes of poor sleep. He is an example of someone with no sleep problems.

NARRATIVE 9—STAN (AB 4/13/10)

Stan was 62 when he completed the questionnaire. Stan says that he has no sleep problems. He goes to bed at 11 P.M., reads for half an hour, turns off the lights, and falls asleep in less than 5 minutes. He wants or needs to arise between 7 and 8 A.M., usually to go to work. About once or twice a month he might wake up between 3 or 4 A.M. and not go back to sleep for about an hour. When he wakes up between 3 and 4 he is not restless; he can lay quite still although wide awake. Rarely, he might wake up at 5:30 A.M. or so and not go back to sleep.

He sleeps on his side and changes sides several times during the night. Although he is aware of turning over, he usually is in a state of semi-consciousness and falls right back to sleep. When he wakes too early once or twice a month, he might feel a bit tired and nap a bit after lunch. He will feel tired or sleepy in the afternoon. Nothing in particular seems to cause his rare nights of sleep loss. He reports that he does have sleep apnea and has a mask, but does not use the mask because it is too restrictive.

He does not take any sleep medications or other sleep aids.

Narrative 21—William (AB 5/13/10)

William did not give his age but is likely to be in the 60s to 70s age range. His sleep habits have never been a serious problem. His bedtime usually is around 10:30 to 11:30 P.M., but time to bed does not give problems. He might read or engage in other activities for 15 minutes before turning off lights, but then falls asleep within 5 minutes. He has no problems falling asleep. He might wake up one or two times during the night, one being a bathroom trip. He likes to get up at 5 A.M., but sometimes wakens at 2:30 to 3:30 A.M. without being able to go back to sleep. His early awakening occurs about 20 times per month.

He indicates no particular causes of early awakenings, except that he mentions night sweats, but does not seem particularly bothered by them. He used to wake up at 6 A.M., but now in later years wakes by 5 A.M. He has no loss of energy when waking early and is alert when arising, but usually needs an afternoon nap. Since he was a teenager, he has always arisen early due to lots of energy and the need to be active. However, in the past 20 years he has arisen earlier at 5 A.M. with some tiredness that is usually relieved by an afternoon nap.

No medications or other sleep aids have been used, but sometimes hot milk or decaffeinated tea in the early evening has helped.

Narrative 35—Martin (AB 7/5/10)

Martin was 77 when he completed the questionnaire. Martin offers that he has no sleep problems, only sleep apnea. He goes to bed between 1 and 2 A.M., does not read but might watch TV in bed for awhile, and then falls asleep within 5 to 10 minutes after turning off the lights. He has no problem with waking up at night and not falling back to sleep. As a retiree, he desires to arise no earlier than 8 to 10 A.M.

His minimal problems of tiredness the next day are caused by sleep apnea, he believes. For the most part, the apnea has been under control by using a Continuous Positive Pressure Airway Pump (CPAP) since 1992.

He has neither tried nor used any other medications or sleep aids than the CPAP.

Men Who Live with Minor Sleep Problems That Are Well Managed

Narrative 37—Bobby (AB 7/30/10)

Bobby was 55 when he completed the questionnaire. He has had sleep problems falling asleep every night for many years. He goes to bed as early as 7 P.M. or stays up late. How long it takes him to go to sleep varies over a wide range. He cannot provide a typical amount of time to go to sleep, or a typical amount of time indulging in activities before going to sleep. If he has something on his mind, he has greater difficulty going to sleep. He needs or desires to get up at 7 A.M., for work or other activities.

One of the causes of wakefulness is his need to urinate frequently during the night. He also suffers from depression and nightmares. During the day, he is alert but tired.

He does not use any medical or self-treatments to help sleep, but when he cannot sleep he spends a lot of time enjoying Facebook. He considers himself a "Facebook addict."

NARRATIVE 1—ARNOLD (AB 4/9/10)

Arnold was 61 when he provided information about his sleep patterns. He usually goes to bed around 11 P.M. to 1 A.M., after reading for one to two hours. Although he is able to go to sleep in 15 minutes to a half-hour after retiring, he often wakes at 2 to 3 A.M. and cannot return to sleep until 4 A.M., needing to get up at 6 to 6:30 to go to work.

The range of his nightly sleep, for most of a month (he estimates 20 to 25 nights out of 30), is thus from about 6¼ to only about 1½ hours. Some of the problem with sleeping is due to some pain, but much of it is due to worries about the security of his job and his financial situation and debts. On his job, he feels tired and unable to work efficiently in the mornings after losing sleep, but recovers and is able to work effectively by 10:30 to 11 A.M. In addition, he has concerns about performance in his part-time volunteer activities, which he hopes to pursue more diligently and successfully upon retirement.

He does not take any sleep medications because he does not want to rely on drugs of any kind. He also does not participate in any other types of sleep therapy. He hopes with faith that his problems will somehow be resolved.

NARRATIVE 39—ROLAND (AB 8/5/10)

Roland was 63 when he completed the questionnaire. He goes to bed between 9:30 and 10:30 P.M. every night, reads or engages in other activities for 15 to 30 minutes, and then turns off the lights. He falls asleep within minutes after turning off the lights. However, he wants to sleep until 5:30 A.M., when he wants or needs to arise, but instead wakes up too early at 2:30 to 3:30 A.M. every morning and cannot return to sleep.

He does not list any of the causes of sleep loss or parasomnias under question 8 of the questionnaire, nor does he list any other causes, so causes *are unknown. His problem with sleep loss is just that he gets tired in the afternoons.*

If he still has four hours left to sleep before wake time, he will take a Benadryl pill. He also uses a sleep mask if waking too early. Also, he gets up and reads or does crossword puzzles when he cannot get back to sleep, because he indicates that he does not like to just toss and turn in bed. He has not sought any medical help nor taken any other remedies. It seems that Roland has primary insomnia, but lives with it and does well.

NARRATIVE 13 — MAURY (AB 4/15/10)

This narrative is written from a questionnaire filled out by the wife of a man who was 71 at the time she completed the questionnaire. Maury and his wife drink one scotch each before going to bed at around 11 P.M. After going to bed, Maury reads for about one hour before turning off the lights and TV. It takes him only about 10 minutes to fall asleep after the lights are turned out. He wakes up once or twice during the night to go to the bathroom, but in the morning hours he can go back to sleep. He describes his morning sleep as "good sleep time." He gets up for the day about 8 to 9 A.M. His sleep problems have been going on for years, but they seem to bother his wife more than him.

He is tired during the day and now takes naps. He never napped at an earlier age. His wife says he has apnea sometimes, especially during early morning hours, although he has not been officially diagnosed. He is also bothered sometimes by seasonal allergies. His doctor has recommended a sleep study, but he has not so far submitted to one. The main problems with his sleep habits are in its effects on his wife. He often snores so loud that she needs to leave and go to another room to sleep. It seems that this apnea causes his poor sleep and his snoring is a serious problem for his wife. She indicates that the problem occurs nightly.

He does take allergy pills and Tylenol PM, as well as eye drops for dry eyes. He has been hesitant to be tested in a sleep study. No permanent therapies or cures have been found.

NARRATIVE 19 — ROLF (AB 5/13/10)

Rolf was 71 at the time of this questionnaire. He usually goes to bed at 10 P.M., reads in bed for 20 to 30 minutes, and then falls asleep within 5 minutes. He usually wants to arise at 6 A.M., but six to eight nights per month he awakens about 3 to 4 A.M. Most of the time if he is tired he goes back to sleep within half an hour. This has been occurring for at least 10 years.

The causes of his inability to go back to sleep after waking early are thinking about things to be done, and trying to resolve some conflict. He often over-commits to work or volunteer activities. He does not have any other causes of sleep loss that he is aware of. The effects of his occasional sleep loss are that he feels tired the next day and has difficulty concentrating on his work. However, if he is standing and teaching a class, or engaging in some other physical activity, he feels all right.

Although he sometimes takes sleeping pills when he wakes up at 3 or 4 A.M., it usually makes him feel groggy the next day and he has trouble writing at his computer or preparing class materials. If he is not tired enough to return to sleep, or is stressed about something, his best bet is to get up and go to work early in the morning; he does this about once or twice a month. He can make up for sleep loss by taking a 45-minute nap in the afternoon, usually between 1 and 3 P.M.

NARRATIVE 11—GERALD (AB 4/14/10)

Gerald was 72 at the time he completed the questionnaire. He takes a sleeping pill every night, because he would otherwise toss and turn and have trouble going to sleep. He goes to bed after midnight; an earlier bedtime does not work for him. He then reads or engages in some other activity for one hour before turning off the lights. The time it takes him to go to sleep varies from night to night. He would like to sleep an hour or two longer than he usually sleeps. He frequently wakes up too early and lies awake for an hour or two. He indicates that he has had these sleep problems for forty years. It is a lifelong problem that sometimes improves and sometimes gets worse. It never totally goes away.

He has no idea what has caused his sleep problems, except that he notes that he has anxiety about sleep and worries that he cannot sleep like the rest of the world; it is especially disconcerting when he is with the family on vacations and cannot sleep like everyone else. Yet, after a night of insufficient sleep, he usually does not have repercussions. When he wakes up during the night, he feels ready to get up and ready for the day, regardless of what the time is. His family seems to have a history of hyperactivity.

Although he has sought medical help many times, usually this help results only in a prescription for sleep medication. Some medications work and some do not. He now takes 10 milligrams of zolpidem each night, which seems to help somewhat. He has also tried massages, hot tubs, cocktails and delaying bedtime. He has never found a cure for his insomnia.

NARRATIVE 18—RALPH (AB 4/17/10)

Ralph was 72 when he completed the questionnaire. He usually goes to bed between 12 and 1 A.M., often tossing and turning with his mind active (but not always). If something surfaces that needs doing, he will sometimes get up and go to his study. After going to bed, he might read or do something else for 1 to 2 hours before turning off the lights. How long it takes him to go to sleep varies; it might be hours. It is an exception when he falls asleep quickly. However, he does not usually wake during the night without being able to go back to sleep. In his retirement he is still very active, but does not get up until about 9 A.M. His sleep problem of not falling to sleep early occurs about half to three-fourths of the time.

He has not listed any particular causes of sleep loss, except that his wife tells him he has apnea. He does not think so, and snores mainly if he sleeps on his back. His insomnia problems have developed over the past few years, and were relatively minor until he had open heart surgery 5 months ago. His problems during the past five months are attributed to post-surgical effects, which caused a fairly minor problem to worsen and not allow him to sleep on his stomach. He does not seem to need much sleep and considers himself a night owl. Sometimes when he is not able to sleep, he goes to his study and surfs the web or does something that needs to be done, perhaps without going back to bed until 4 A.M. or even later. The next day he feels fine, getting up by 10 or 10:30 and not usually needing a nap. He might sometimes feel drowsy in late afternoon and take a nap for an hour or so. By the end of dinner, he is fully awake again, whether he has taken a nap or not.

He did not list any of the usual causes of sleep loss, nor has he tried any medications or other sleep aids. He continues to lead an active life in his professional and volunteer pursuits. He lives well with whatever insomnia he might have.

Men Who Have Concerns or Difficulties with Sleep Problems

NARRATIVE 14—ANTHONY (AB 4/15/10)

Anthony was 19 when he completed the questionnaire. He goes to bed about 10 P.M. to 12 A.M. and wakes between 6 to 9 A.M. He usually reads or engages in other activities about 30 minutes to two hours before turning off the lights. After he turns off lights, he has bursts of energy and racing thoughts that at first keep him awake. It takes him between about 30 minutes to two hours to fall asleep. From 1 to 5 A.M. he awakens about four times a night. When he wakes between 4 and 6 A.M., it takes him about 30 minutes to fall asleep. He has these sleep problems about 25 out of 30 nights, and they have lasted for years.

Causes of his sleepless nights include bad work schedules and sleep during the day that takes away tiredness and the need for sleep at night. He also lists night sweats, anxiety, and nightmares as causes of sleep loss.

He has taken trazodone to help himself fall asleep, but although it might help him fall asleep he does not stay asleep. He has found no effective cures.

NARRATIVE 34—PATRICK (AB 7/3/10)

Patrick was 59 when he completed the questionnaire. For about four to five years, Patrick has had problems about every night with some loss of sleep and a feeling of tiredness during the day. At some point he found himself falling asleep at the wheel at traffic light stops and consulted a neurologist. He has no problem falling asleep at night, regardless of when he goes to sleep. He usually goes to bed between 10 and 11 P.M., reads or engages in other activities for about 20 minutes before turning off the lights, and then falls asleep within about 25 minutes. Usually a couple of times a week he will wake up between 2 and 3 A.M. before setting his alarm. He wants to get up between 4 and 5 A.M. to prepare for going to work, depending on what time he gets to bed. He usually cannot go back to sleep once he wakes up, but this had occurred long before he had felt he had any sleep problems. Usually a couple of times a week he wakes up an hour before his alarm is set to go off.

Causes of his sleep loss or light sleep have been periodic limb movement disorder (PLMD), slight apnea, and arm pain due to carpal tunnel syndrome. At one point after taking a prescription, his PLMD turned into restless leg syndrome, at which point he could not sleep at all. His prescription was changed and things improved for awhile. The effects of his sleep problems have been loss of energy during the day on his job or elsewhere, and sleepiness while driving.

He has not taken any over-the-counter sleep aids or other self-help sleep regimes. When his problem became serious, he was sent to a neurologist by his family doctor. A sleep study revealed that he had mild sleep apnea, heavy snoring, and PLMD. The neurologist did not think the mild sleep apnea was serious. The first medication the neurologist prescribed to improve his sleep, along with Provigil to aid daytime attentiveness, caused the restless leg syndrome and was replaced by Neurontin. Then, his sleep became normal for awhile. About one to one and a half years later his sleep was not as refreshing; his neurologist put him on one dose, and then a greater dose, of imipramine, but this did not help much. He is planning another visit soon to the neurologist.

Observations from the Narratives

Even in this small sample taken as convenient, with no sampling design planned to represent any specific population, the vast majority of sleep patterns and problems presented in other chapters—symptoms, causes, effects, and attempted treatments or therapies—are seen to be present in the persons sampled. This is found to parallel the experience of Hite: the myriad of factors in human sexuality were found even in her first sample of only 45 women, which launched her first bestseller.[2] Her findings from this sample were essentially confirmed in her more exhaustive study using a sample of 3,000. We mention this parallel because many statisticians will think that little information on fractions of persons in several categories would be forthcoming from such a limited population sample.

Neubauer,[3] after defining insomnia as requiring the two experiences of sleep loss and significant suffering afterward, lists 10 complaints to illustrate the many variations of experience described to therapists. These complaints are paraphrased from his book as follows:

1. I take too long to fall asleep at night.
2. I awaken through the night, like every hour.
3. I never get deep sleep anymore, and am always in a twilight state.
4. I have not slept in months.
5. I wake up too early and cannot get back to sleep.
6. I cannot shut off my mind at night.
7. I drag myself out of bed in the morning because my sleep is so bad.
8. I never feel rested.
9. I am fatigued all day.
10. I could not nap even if my life depended on it.

Neubauer, a clinical psychiatrist in the Johns Hopkins Sleep Disorders Center as well as a research scientist, relates the first six items to a sense of very light sleep and the complaints about initiating and maintaining sleep. The last four items are the negative daytime symptoms of the sleep loss. It is also evident that items 7 to 9 would be strongly correlated with each other; they would not be independent.

Neubauer also recognizes that shift work will alter the sleep cycle, as indicated by our friend in regard to native inhabitants of our Eastern Shore communities. Related to this, he also points out that some problems result from our cultural expectation in the United States that we must get eight hours' sleep during the night; he devotes his book mainly to the United States population.

Looking over the narratives of the limited sample of questionnaire responders, we can see that all of the ten complaints listed by Neubauer are present somewhere among the individuals in our sample, usually with one or more of the Neubauer's first six sleep problems occurring in the first paragraph of a narrative being correlated with the complaints 7 to 10 in the second paragraph, respectively.

It is also interesting to the authors, as observed in Chapter 3, that Allen has experienced complaints 1 to 9 on many nights and days, but not complaint 10, while Phyllis has experienced all of items 1 through 10.

For those who might now want to read some narratives of personal interest, the narratives are listed below, with the specific complaint numbers of Neubauer to identify complaints that might be of interest to the reader. (See if you match some of them and if they are in your category.)

- In Narrative 1, Arnold exhibits complaint 5 frequently and suffers from complaints 7 to 9 to a large degree; however, he does indicate that he recovers some energy in later morning, so 8 and 9 are restricted mainly to early morning.
- In Narrative 2, Beth has complaints 2, 5, and 8, although 2 and 5 occur only about 5 nights per month.
- In Narrative 3, Donna occasionally has complaints 5 and 9. She states she lacks focus but is energetic after losing sleep, but she can take naps.
- In Narrative 4, Bunny has no complaints, even if she needs to arise to go to the bathroom.
- In Narrative 5, Dolly occasionally has complaints 5 and 8 or 9. They occur only a few times a month now in her retirement.
- In Narrative 6, Lonnie is similar to Narrative 4. Only rarely does she feel tired after losing some sleep. If she complained, she might be considered a very infrequent 8. She does not have a sleep problem.
- In Narrative 7, Sherry has complaints similar to 2, 5, and 8, especially in later years after menstruation.
- In Narrative 8, Ellen has complaints similar to 2, 5, 8, and 9.
- In Narrative 9, Stan feels that he has no sleep problems. Only once or twice a month will he have complaints 5 and 8 (only temporarily; he soon regains energy).
- In Narrative 10, Carla has sleep problems about half of any month, involving complaints 5, and 8 or 9.
- In Narrative 11, Gerald sometimes has complaint 5 but does not let it bother him. He has energy whenever he is awake.

- In Narrative 12, Elise has sleep problems 7 to 12 times a month, her complaints being 5 and 9.
- In Narrative 13, Maury's sleep problems bother mainly his wife, with complaints 2 and 3 every night.
- In Narrative 14, Anthony frequently has complaints 2, 5, 6, and also 8 during days when he cannot nap.
- In Narrative 15, Marian has sleep loss 8 to 10 nights per month that involve complaints 1, 2, 5, and 8.
- In Narrative 16, Bernadette has complaints about sleep that fall into numbers 1, 5, and 6. However, although she is concerned about her sleep loss, she has only complaint 8 when arising and does not feel tired during the day. She has memory loss but attributes it to aging rather than sleep loss.
- In Narrative 17, Shannon has complaints 1 and sometimes 5, but does not express complaints 7 through 10 but indicates problems with anxiety, depression, and fibromyalgia. Perhaps if she were not retired, these latter problems would be expressed as tiredness and fatigues at work.
- In Narrative 18, Ralph has complaints 1, 5, and 6 about sleep, but in his retirement is not concerned about tiredness or fatigue. After a nap, he is energetic in performing his activities and writings.
- In Narrative 19, Rolf has complaint 5 about six to eight nights per month, and sometimes complaint 8, but if he is busy or lecturing he becomes alert. Sometimes if he awakens too early and cannot get back to sleep, he will get up and write or prepare lectures.
- In Narrative 20, Rena has complaint 5 about eight times a month, followed by complaint 8 that is now subdued after retirement.
- In Narrative 21, William has complaint 5 about 20 times a month and complaint 8, which can be alleviated by a nap.
- In Narrative 22, June has complaints 5 and 8 only seven or eight times a month.
- In Narrative 23, Constance has no trouble falling asleep or sleeping, except that she has complaint 8 when her schedule does not allow her to complete her sleep.
- In Narrative 24, Alice has no sleep problems most of the time, but very occasionally has complaint 2 and some degree of complaint 8 the next day.
- In Narrative 25, Kevin is in college and has a sleep complaint 5 only about once a month. However, he is an energetic person and feels fine the next day.

- In Narrative 26, Evelyn is in college and also works nights. She has sleep problems every night because she must stay up late into the wee hours of the morning. However, sometimes her complaint is number 5. She sometimes has complaint 7 but has no other complaints because she feels she must accept what she needs to do.
- In Narrative 27, Ethel has sleep problem 1 only twice a month but sleep complaint 5 often, with complaint 8 and 9 after sleep loss.
- In Narrative 28, Neena has complaint 1 about half the time and complaint 5 more often. Sleep loss is often followed by complaint 8, except that sometimes she still feels great even after little sleep.
- In Narrative 29, Marilyn often has number 1, but would not call it a complaint. She accepts sleep as it comes, and is alert day and night. She could not be considered to have insomnia.
- In Narrative 30, Lorena indicates she has no sleep problems. Although she occasionally does not get enough sleep and feels somewhat tired the next day, she has none of the complaints.
- In Narrative 31, Karen, for about four nights per month, has complaints 5 or 6, which results in complaints 8 or 9 on those days. She attributes her problems to her erratic college schedule. Her sleep has improved now that class is over.
- In Narrative 32, Esther has problem 5 about once or twice a month, resulting in 8 the next day. However, she attributes the problem to college stresses and does not consider that she has any sleep problems.
- In Narrative 33, Darlene often has complaint 5, attributable to 6, but lives with insomnia in her retirement, without needing to wake up or get up at any time.
- In Narrative 34, Patrick for the past five years has had complaint 5, resulting in complaints 8 and 9, falling asleep at traffic lights on the way home from work. He is now seeking further changes in medications.
- In Narrative 35, Martin has had no sleep problems since using oxygen from a CPAP in 1992. He is retired now and can adjust to any tiredness that sometimes results.
- In Narrative 36, Libby has complaint 5 about three times a week. She feels tired when arising but alert during work until late afternoon when she has complaint 8.
- In Narrative 37, Bobby has had all sleep complaints 1 through 6 for many years, and effects 7 to 9 much of the time, but not 10. He has lived with these symptoms and carried on with life, without attempting medical or

self-treatments. Therefore, he has been put into the "living with insomnia" middle category of men.

- In Narrative 38, Joleen has had symptom 5 only occasionally and manages it well. She has no sleep problems.
- In Narrative 39, Roland has only symptom 5 and symptom 8 in the afternoon. He seems to have primary insomnia but lives well with it.
- In Narrative 40, Ramsey has no sleep complaints at all. He is rare.
- In Narrative 41, Millie has sleep complaints only 2 to 3 times a month. She has only symptom 7 on these occasions, and manages her sleep problems so well that she provides the best example of good sleep hygiene and habits encountered so far.
- In Narrative 42, Bess has sleep complaints every night and they affect her life. She has symptoms 2, 3, 4, 5, 6, 7, 8, 9, and 10.

Use of Narratives to Compare Them with Your Own Sleep Patterns

Reading these abbreviated descriptions of sleep problems, related to Neubauer's ten complaints, the reader might find similar experiences to his own in one or more narratives. In this way, he might also find suggestions that are helpful in understanding his own sleep problems and possible remedies tried by others. This is one reason that all narratives from our sample have been placed together in this chapter. The other reason is that we can then refer back to these narratives by number and sex when we use them to make a point or comparison, and the reader may easily find them if he desires to examine them for additional perspectives.

Other observations from these narratives derived from questionnaires respond to the questions in the last paragraph of Chapter 3:

It is interesting that all of the sleep problems experienced by the authors, as described in Chapter 3, do appear in the narratives of this chapter. However, the authors' experiences in Chapter 3 have not been derived from the standard questionnaires presented to participants, and are not included in the scenarios of this chapter. The authors' descriptions of their own sleep experiences would be even more subjective than the narratives descriptions presented in this chapter. The placement of the narratives in this chapter, for each sex, according to no insomnia, living with insomnia, or insomnia of serious concern, is of course somewhat subjective because of the need to decide the indicated seriousness of the sleep loss in each case. However, the proportion of cases in each category seem to approximate those found in larger studies. The number of cases of men and women that we have placed in the serious insomnia categories turns out to be consistent with the 10 to 15 percent serious cases quoted by Neubauer from the literature.[4]

Also subjective can be the estimates of amount of sleep loss provided by participants. As Neubauer points out, "there is a surprisingly weak correspondence" between the amounts of sleep loss reported by, and the objective measurements of sleep loss obtained from, respective participants in sleep laboratories.[5]

An additional insight is that many of the sleep questionnaire respondents in the middle category, those who "live with" insomnia, both men and women, do not worry excessively about their sleep and manage to enjoy active and productive lives despite sleep loss. This is similar to the experiences of Allen as presented in Chapter 3, where he describes in his early life the need to avoid worry about sleep and plow on with his work and life obligations, tired the next day or not. In particular, we see that the responders of college age have had similar necessary learning experiences. A further observation appears: even in this small sample, women seem to more frequently suffer from insomnia, as indicated in previous chapters and due to the causes presented before.

An Insomnia Card Game for Fun and Finding You Are Not Alone

This card game can be played by a couple, or played solitaire by a single person dealing cards to an imaginary partner. The dealing can be done as many times as the couple desires, until they feel satisfied they have experienced the range of sleep problems, habits, or effects pertinent to each of them; or until they get bored. They can also read to each other and discuss between deals the pertinent narratives numbered on their draws, if they want to enhance their appreciation of problems and solutions of others in comparison with their own.

Here is how the game is played:

1. On the back of each card in a deck, use a soft permanent marker to write the numbers 1 in sequence, up to 52, or fewer if desired. This will not destroy the deck.

2. Before each deal, each partner selects ahead of time and writes down three of the ten complaints listed by Neubauer that he or she has selected of personal interest.

3. Then, the cards are shuffled and five cards (or however many is desired) are dealt to each player.

4. Each player compares the numbers of the complaints he or she selected to the numbers of the complaints of the numbered responders on his or her respective card.

5. The person with the least number of times the complaints selected beforehand are found in the narratives of the numbered individuals on his or her cards WINS THE GAME! (Now, this does not mean I am recommending gambling for money.)

NOTE: If you do not like this game the way I (Allen) designed it, make one up yourself! (Don't blame Phyllis.)

Sexual Factors

One important set of factors that can enhance or detract from healthy sleep does *not* appear explicitly in these questionnaires. Depending on situations and personal preferences, matters of sexual and family love, or conflict, can have positive or negative effects on sleep. At the beginning, the authors decided that this book could not deal in detail with this complex subject. Questionnaires involving explicit questions about sex might be difficult to circulate with an expectation of responses in the closed communities available to the authors. It is evident that this was probably a good decision, because none of the respondents to the questionnaires volunteered to present any matters of sexual experience in their responses about causes or effects of lack of sleep, or enhancement of sleep.

Because matters of sexual desire, satisfaction, or frustration can have serious affects on sleep patterns, the authors recommend to readers that if any sexual matters seriously affect sleep or life circumstances, those involved should consult professional physicians or therapists who specialize in sex counseling. This is particularly important if those involved cannot find resolution of such problems through the vast book and article literature always available to the public, in stores or on the internet. A small, but likely helpful, set of books on human sexuality that can provide insights related to healthy sleep will be included in the bibliography. As with any problem, improved understanding of the problem and possible solutions can go a long way toward resolving relational or sexual frustrations that affect sleep. Private conversations with trusted friends, counselors, or physicians can help along with reading to understand the nature and remedies for sleeplessness associated with relational or sexual frustrations.

CHAPTER 7

Parasomnias

Parasomnias are unusual, sometimes strange, sleep disorders that might or might not cause insomnia. Such sleep disorders are generally not a problem of too little sleep, but the strange behaviors can be disturbing to the person exhibiting such actions, to his or her partner, or to other family members. One doesn't hear about these disorders too often. I (Phyllis), for one, had not heard of the term "parasomnia," except, of course, sleep talking and sleepwalking, until I started reading about them for this book.

According to Michael J. Breus, PhD., a diplomate of the American Board of Sleep Medicine, "A parasomnia is a classification of sleep disorder where people can do some pretty complicated behaviors in their sleep."[1] About 10 percent of adults suffer from some sort of parasomnia.[2] There are several sleep disorders that are classified as parasomnias that will be explored in this chapter. The cause of most of these conditions is unknown, but there may be a genetic connection, since some of these disorders tend to run in families.

Parasomnias have been described in the *International Classification of Sleep Disorders* (ICSD) as, "undesirable physical events or experiences occurring during sleep transition, on arousal from sleep, or while sleeping." Some are more common in children, but they usually do not persist into adulthood.[3] Parasomnias are classified according to the time of night and/or the stage of sleep in which episodes occur. These classifications are sleep-onset (hypnagogic) parasomnias, disorders of arousal, disorders associated with REM sleep, and others that occur at various times during the sleep cycle. Also, some parasomnias are associated with medical or psychiatric disorders.

Hypnagogic Parasomnias (sleep-onset)

The hypnagogic disorders are those that occur upon falling asleep or early in the sleep cycle. *Hypnagogic images* or sensations are common while falling asleep, but usually not remembered unless the person awakens at that time. These are of little consequence. *Sleep starts* are fleeting sensory motor sensations as simple as someone's leg or knee jerking or the feeling of falling. These are not disturbing and of little or no consequence. I (Phyllis) have experienced both of these events from time to time and thought nothing of it. I thought that I had been dreaming.

Hypnagogic hallucinations also occur in the minutes before falling asleep or soon after. These can be more frightening than fleeting images. These are not normal, because dreaming normally doesn't happen until about ninety minutes into the sleep cycle. The visual images are very vivid, such as changes in shape, size, or color of familiar objects in the bedroom. These images are not remembered unless the person wakes up. Hypnagogic hallucinations are also associated with other sleep disorders, such as narcolepsy, sleepwalking, sleep terrors, and REM behavior disorders, which will be discussed later in this chapter. These symptoms also occur in people who are severely sleep-deprived, such as truck drivers who are traveling long distances.[4]

Sleep Paralysis is another sleep-onset disorder. As mentioned earlier, voluntary muscles of the arms and legs are temporarily paralyzed in REM sleep. When paralysis occurs early in the sleep cycle—in non–REM sleep—it is not a normal occurrence. When it does occur, it generally lasts only a few seconds to several minutes. However, it can be frightening if the person wakes up and cannot move. It stops on its own or by being touched or spoken to by the parent or bed partner.[5]

This disorder can occur on transition from wakefulness to sleep or from sleep to wakening. Basically, the body is asleep, but the brain is awake. Dr. Schenck describes this disorder as "REM sleep and its parts are trying to invade wakefulness and show up on the scene as soon as possible once the person has fallen asleep, or persist when the person is awakening...."[6] Episodes usually last only briefly or a few minutes. Sleep paralysis occurs in 0.05 percent of the U.S. population. It is believed to be caused by a deficiency in a brain chemical, called hypocretin, which is normally located in the major brain center that regulates the sleep-awake cycle. There may be a genetic predisposition to this disorder. Sleep paralysis is also a symptom of narcolepsy. It can also be accompanied by hallucinations.[7] There are medications that are effective in treating this disorder.

Disorders of Arousal

These parasomnias occur early in the night during deep, delta stage sleep. These are non–REM disorders. People troubled with these disorders don't completely arouse from sleep, but tend to drift between sleep and wakefulness. Sleepwalking is probably the most common of this group of sleep disorders.

Sleepwalking, also known as somnambulism, originates during deep sleep, soon after falling asleep or in the early part of the sleep cycle. It is more common in children and is generally outgrown by adolescence. In some cases, it continues into adulthood or can be first expressed during adulthood.

There are a range of behaviors among sleepwalkers. For example, a person might just sit up in bed. Others get out of bed and walk around. They might perform complex behaviors. There are extreme cases in which individuals actually leave their houses and walk around outside, or even get in their cars and drive somewhere. A young marine told us about a buddy who was a sleepwalker and remembered on one occasion that this man did drive while sleeping. There have also been instances where an individual might engage in inappropriate behavior, such as urinating in a closet. If the person has to urinate, the closet may be mistaken for the bathroom. Allen told me this happened to him as a child (as related in his personal story in Chapter 3).

On another occasion, Allen believes that he had an experience similar to driving while sleeping. He wants to relate the experience here:

Soon after the Three Mile Island nuclear accident in 1979, Dr. Petr Beckman asked me (Allen) to take his place on a Miami TV show to debate Dr. George Wald about the safety of nuclear power. Dr. Beckman had needed to finish grading student papers. Although I had a bad cold with a sore throat, I agreed to sit in on this Saturday night Miami debate show. Dr. Beckman had already done so much, publishing a book and newsletter revealing the true safety aspects of nuclear energy compared to other sources. I could not refuse this simple request. On Saturday evening before the show, I had a couple of martinis to soothe my throat. On the Sunday after the show, the cold was worse, so I took a couple of Coricidin pills at lunch, and had another couple of drinks. After visiting my lawyer cousin Maury, I then drove to another part of Miami and visited Maury's sister and husband. Before I left the second visit for the airport, the sister's husband, knowing of my sore throat and being a pharmacist, offered another medication: a glass with about 6 ounces of vodka "for the road." I, always having been able to hold a number of drinks previously and still drive safely, chug-a-lugged the glass of whiskey, and headed for the Miami airport, where I had never driven to before from this location. I remember looking at a map before starting to drive. The next thing I was aware of was waking up face down, fully clothed, on a bed at the airport motel. I wondered what happened to my rental car, and then vaguely remembered giving a tip to an airport porter to turn the car in. It was as if the porter had appeared in a dream. Next, I looked at my watch—an ordinary watch. It read just a short hour or so after the time in the afternoon that I had planned to arrive at the airport for an afternoon flight back to Washington, D.C. I quickly arose fulled clothed in a suit with vest, thinking there was no time to waste in catching my afternoon flight. I dashed from the hotel room with my bag to the airport and my airline's ticket and check-in counters. When I arrived at the check-in counters, the airport seemed empty. One agent was at the counter in the otherwise rather vacant area. I asked the man what happened to my flight. The man looked at my ticket and said, "Dr. Brodsky, your plane left yesterday! It is now 5 A.M. on Monday morning!" Apparently, all of the whisky and Coricidin were very effective in putting me to sleep for about 12 hours, completely clothed in my suit. The porter to whom I left my car must have been an honest, caring man who had helped me to this room. It is just a bit frightening that my drinks and medication had put me to sleep while I was driving in a route strange to me. Yet, I must somehow have driven safely. I assume that this was a case where, although initiated by too much alcohol and medicine, I was *driving in my sleep*. Yet, one remaining mystery is how my cheap watch knew it should stop at the same time I was induced to sleep. Is there an undiscovered force communicating between people and their wrist watches? Or, was some higher authority watching over me and sending a message? After I reset the watch, it continued to work fine. After this experience, I have never again chug-a-lugged strong drinks; I just sip slowly on an ounce at a time. Now I know that I do have limits. I drink alcohol now only in moderation.

Back again to Phyllis and sleepwalking. Although sleepwalking is a non–REM parasomnia, I (Phyllis) remember dreaming that "I had to get home," in the story I revealed in Chapter 3. I can't explain this. Some sleepwalkers may even rearrange furniture or fix something to eat. (There is also a "sleep eaters" parasomnia—included later in this chapter). Needless to say, the consequences of these more extreme behaviors could be dangerous to the inflicted person or to others.

People who are observed sleepwalking act as if they are awake, but will not respond to other people around them. Although asleep, the person's eyes are open, but have a glassy-eyed and confused look. While engaging in these complex behaviors, the person remains asleep and does not remember the episode upon awakening. However, if they are awakened during the episode, they might remember. The prevalence of sleepwalking is about 1 to 15 percent of the general population, but much higher in children.[8] According to Dr. Schlenck, in his book, *Sleep*, 17 percent of children between the ages of 4 and 12 years have had one or more sleepwalking episodes.[9]

It is interesting that, while sleepwalking, people are not dreaming. Sleepwalking tends to run in families; so there may be a genetic basis. Episodes can be triggered by severe sleep deprivation, some medications, or alcohol. Dr. Dement, in his book, *The Promise of Sleep*, points out that children begin to give up their daytime naps at about four years of age, when sleepwalking tends to emerge. When the children give up their naps, they initially become sleep deprived. Dr. Dement explains that brain wave recordings show that sleepwalkers pass back and forth between sleep and wakefulness. They wake up just enough that the most primitive parts of the brain are working, but not the cognitive parts.[10]

If you witness a family member sleepwalking, it is best not to wake him or her up, unless he or she is in potential danger, such as falling down steps, falling out of a window, or headed out the door. Try gently guiding him or her back to bed. If it appears danger is eminent, then the person has to be awakened by gentle touching and calling his or her name.

Parents of children who sleepwalk are usually awake since episodes generally occur early in the sleep cycle. Children's bedrooms should be kept child-proof—that is, all sharp and fragile items should be out of reach. Doors and windows should be locked and a gate fastened on top of staircases. It is also obvious that the child should not sleep in a bunk bed.[11] Children generally grow out of this disorder, but it can continue onto adulthood. If the consequences of sleepwalking pose risks, then the disorder should be treated.

If there are underlying causes, such as sleep deprivation, migraine headaches, seizure disorders, previous head injury, fever, or obstructive sleep apnea, these conditions should be evaluated and treated. A large percentage of sleepwalkers have obstructive sleep apnea or other breathing disorders. There is a genetic basis in 65 percent of sleepwalkers.[12] This cannot be changed, but other known causative conditions should be corrected.

Clonazepam (Klonopin) is an effective drug in the treatment of sleepwalking and other parasomnias.[13] This drug is in the family of benzodiazepines. The well-known drug Valium falls in this class of drugs, of which the main actions are anti-anxiety and anti-convulsant. Some of these drugs also have hypnotic (sleep-inducing) effects. Clonazepam has low abuse potential and negligible risks. This medication seems to decrease the brain's response to environmental stimuli, including the stimuli from dreams.[14]

Sleep Terrors also referred to as night terrors, occur during non–REM sleep, during the early stages of sleep. They are distinct from nightmares. The episodes are frightening to observers (parents or bed partner), but not remembered by the sleeper. The episode begins with the person rising up in bed, seemingly out of deep sleep, in a seemingly terrified state, screaming. Strangely, these night terrors are not frightening for the child, but certainly can be initially frightening for a parent, sleep partner, or other person in the home. (In Chapter 3, Allen has indicated his concern when I have suddenly screamed at night in my sleep, not remembering it on awakening the next morning.) In the laboratory, brain recordings indicate that the person is passing back and forth between sleep and wakefulness.[15]

Sleep terrors are more prevalent in children ages 3 to 12 years, but do sometimes begin in adulthood. Episodes only last a few minutes, sometimes a little longer. There is no known underlying psychiatric disorder or other cause. It can be attributed to sudden impulses in the brain that trigger a hyperarousal state, in which the person's heart rate, respiratory rate, and blood pressure temporarily increase. The person is also observed sweating. Stress can trigger—not cause—an episode. There may also be a genetic predisposition. Sometimes sleep terrors are associated with sleepwalking. If the person suddenly jumps out of bed, seemingly in terror, they then have both conditions.[16]

There is no particular treatment for children. Parents should just comfort them by gently cuddling them in their arms and speaking softly. Practice of good sleep hygiene, such as assuming regular sleep schedules, and, for adults, avoiding alcohol and caffeine beverages in the evening, helps to decrease the occurrence of these episodes. It is also helpful to determine any underlying precipitating factors, such as sleep deprivation, other sleep disorders, or medical problems that trigger sleep terrors. Once underlying disorders are diagnosed, they can be treated.[17]

Confusional arousals are similar to night terrors. They are seen mostly in young children, but can also occur in adults. During an episode of confusion, the person seems to be awake, confused, and distressed, but is actually asleep.[18] This disorder typically occurs on arousal from deep sleep early in the night and is characterized by the inertia most people experience on arising from sound sleep. They generally don't remember recent happenings and respond slowly to questions or demands. It is not an unusual occurrence, and probably should not even be classified as a "disorder."[19]

Sleep-Related Eating Disorder (SRED) is another strange phenomenon that can occur during sleep. This disorder is another non–REM parasomnia. It occurs during sleep walking (obviously). The person affected with this disorder had to get out of bed and walk to the kitchen, which is the logical place to find food. Although SRED is classified as a non–REM disorder, it can happen at any time during the night. Such afflicted persons are asleep and don't remember the episodes, but they do leave evidence, such as a messy kitchen or crumbs in their bed. The worst part is that they tend to gain weight. There is also risk of injury, which could occur by banging into walls, chairs, the refrigerator, or other objects, and they might even cut themselves while slicing food. They might also have dental problems from eating a lot of sweets, or gnawing on frozen foods. People with this disorder often make a beeline for the kitchen several times a night and binge on sweet, high-calorie foods.[20]

For the most part, people with this disorder have no memory of these events; others have some awareness, but might have no control of what the sleeping eater is doing. The sleep-eater's compulsion to eat is not related to hunger, pain, or health problems. This disorder affects women more than men. The consequences are enormous—weight gain and obesity, feeling of bloating in the morning, disruptive sleep, and feeling exhausted the following day. It can also induce or aggravate health problems, such as diabetes, hypertension, high cholesterol, heart problems, and dental problems.[21]

People who have sleep disorders such as restless leg syndrome, obstructive sleep apnea, a history of binge eating, or a family history of parasomnias are at risk for developing this strange parasomnia. Also, people who have stopped abusing drugs or alcohol are at risk. Some medications, such as tricyclic antidepressants, and Ambien, the most commonly prescribed sleep medication at the present time, can potentially trigger sleep-eating binges.[22]

Abnormal Sleepsex (also referred to as "Sexsomnia") is a fairly recent discovery. It is another bizarre, recently defined parasomnia, in which the person acts out various aggressive sexual behaviors, such as sexual verbalizations, masturbation, fondling his bed partner, or, on occasion, forced intercourse, and yet be sound asleep. They do not remember any of the behaviors upon awakening and are not normally sexually aggressive. Sleepsex is a non–REM sleep disorder. Dr. Schenck, in his 2007 book, *Sleep*, exclaimed that after searching the literature, he found 31 documented cases, 80 percent of who were men in their early thirties. These men also suffered from confusional arousals and sleepwalking.[23]

Most people who exhibit such behaviors are also known sleepwalkers. The aggressive sexual behaviors they exhibit while sleeping are not the way they normally behave when awake. Their abnormal sexual behaviors while sleeping can be exacerbated by poor quality or quantity of sleep, sleep deprivation, alcohol consumption, and sleep apnea.[24]

The disorder is difficult to diagnose and can result in relationship problems and legal ramifications. For instance, the afflicted person could be accused of engaging in forced sex, could lose trust from his partner, and cause his partner pain and bruising. The partner may find it hard to believe that the behaviors are unintended. The causes of the disorder are not known. It seems that something triggers the person to arouse out of a deep sleep into a quasi-awake state, unleashing primitive and confused behaviors. There is hope for this condition. It can be effectively treated with the drug clonazepam (Klonopin), which is effective in 90 percent of cases.[25]

Parasomnias Associated with REM Sleep

In review, REM sleep takes place following stages 3 and 4 (slow wave, deep sleep). People dream during REM sleep, a time when their voluntary muscles are temporarily paralyzed. (The muscles that control breathing, heart, and other "autonomic" functions are not paralyzed—or the person would be in deep trouble.) The other interesting part of REM sleep is that men's penises become erect, as explained earlier.

REM sleep disorders are characterized by vivid dreaming, and also include nightmares, more frequent awakenings than other parasomnias, and potential violent behaviors. These disorders result in sleep disruption and greater difficulty falling back to sleep. The underlying pathology of these disorders is a disturbance in the brainstem mechanism that normally inhibits nerve transmission to the motor center in the cortex. Under normal conditions, this inhibition of nerve transmission inhibits movement.[26] As a result, the person is able to move about, walk, and exhibit various activities that occur in these abnormal sleep patterns. What causes this brain disturbance is a mystery.

Nightmares are different from night terrors. Whereas sleep terrors occur early during slow-wave, non–REM sleep, nightmares occur in the middle of the night, or later, during REM sleep. Generally, the person is aroused from the nightmare.

Nightmares occur when the person has a disturbing or frightening dream. If the person then wakes up screaming, he or she generally becomes fully awake and immediately remembers the dream. There is either no obvious reason that a nightmare occurs; sometimes it might follow after the person had been watching a disturbing movie or television program prior to going to sleep. Persistent nightmares can be caused by a previous frightening experience or underlying cause, such as post-traumatic stress disorder.[27] There also might be no obvious reason that nightmares happen. As I described in Chapter 3, I had recurring nightmares as a child. I still have nightmares on occasion and do frequently remember what I had been dreaming. However, the memory is vague and quickly forgotten. I've frightened my husband on several occasions.

REM Behavioral Disorder (RBD) is a more serious form of nightmare. Dreams become nightmares and there is absence of paralysis, which is otherwise a normal happening during REM sleep. Dreams are a mental activity, but in RBD, the person's dreams are actually acted out. This disorder is more common in men, but occasionally occurs in women and children. The person can physically move his or her arms and legs. He or she might talk, shout, scream, or even hit or kick a bed partner, causing injury to self or bed partner. Different from ordinary dreams or nightmares, in RBD, dreams are acted out and remembered.[28]

The violent activity is related to terrified dreams of being attacked by someone unknown or some animal. The dreams are horrible. About 90 percent of those afflicted are men. The disorder appears to be more common in people who have had a brain injury or infection earlier in their lives. It can also be a rare adverse effect from certain antidepressant medications.[29] RBD usually affects people over 50 years of age who have never been violent or aggressive while awake. This disturbance can also be a consequence of Parkinson's disease. Both Parkinson's disease and RBD have disruptions of neurochemicals in the same area of the brain. Normally, nerve messages in that area of the brain block movement of the limbs during REM sleep; this doesn't happen in RBD.[30] This disorder is treated with clonazepam, which is effective 90 percent of the time. Anti-depressant medications or melatonin have also been shown to be effective in reducing violent behavior in people with RBD.[31]

Other Parasomnias Occurring at Various Times of the Night

Sleep talking is a common occurrence. It can at occur any age, and any time during the sleep cycle. The person is not aware of talking, unless he or she awakens during the episode. I (Phyllis) do it frequently. It doesn't bother me in the least; but it sure interests my husband when he is awake. (He thinks he might learn some of my secrets, so he turns in my direction if he is awake; but I mostly mumble—so he tells me—and he can't understand what I'm saying.) Sometimes I wake up for a brief minute and remember what I had been dreaming. If he knows I am awake, he might ask what I have been dreaming. Usually, I do not tell him because I do not remember. Anyway, it is none of his business, so I try to go back to sleep.

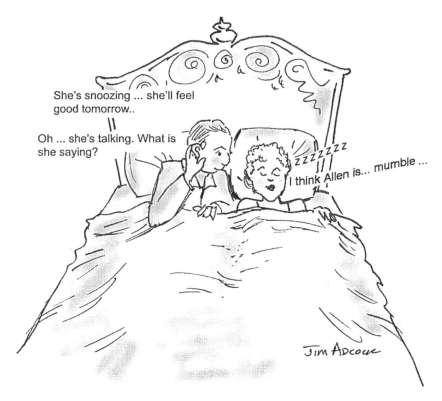

Exhibit 2. Allen listening in on Phyllis's Sleep Talk. Allen says, "Sometimes I am happy to hear her snoozing, but then she mumbles something in her sleep, and I try to spy on her dreams."

Sleep talking can occur concurrently with other sleep disorders, such as sleep terror, confusional arousals, and other REM sleep disorders. It can be precipitated by stress, sleep deprivation, alcohol, and depression. The mutterings make no sense, but may relate to past experiences that no longer have meaning or reason.[32]

Narcolepsy

Narcolepsy does not fall into any of the above categories of sleep disorders. It is an unusual neurological disorder, characterized by extreme sleepiness during the day. It is not a psychological or psychotic disorder. Those afflicted can't help falling asleep spontaneously for short periods of time—

about 15 minutes or longer—occurring about every three to four hours throughout the day. These "sleep attacks" can occur after eating, while conversing with others, while driving, or while performing any activity.[33] People who have this disorder also have poor sleep quality at night.

Narcolepsy tends to run in families. There is a reduced amount of a specific neurotransmitter (brain chemical) called hypocretin, in the part of the brain that regulates sleep. It is not known why there is a deficit of this important neurotransmitter. There are other distinct manifestations of this disorder, which constitute the four defining symptoms of narcolepsy: daytime sleep attacks, sleep paralysis, hypnagogic hallucinations, and cataplexy.

Sleep attacks are described above. *Sleep paralysis* is a state in which the person is unable to move his or her limbs and is even unable to talk when falling asleep or waking up. People have reported being fully awake and aware during these episodes, but not being able to move or talk. These happenings can be terrifying.

A third symptom is the occurrence of *hypnagogic hallucinations*, in which the person has very vivid dreams upon falling asleep or waking up. During these episodes, the person immediately goes into REM sleep as soon as he or she falls asleep again.[34]

Cataplexy is a syndrome in which sufferers may experience sudden episodes of severe muscle weakness, which can be triggered by a strong emotional reaction, such as surprise, laughter, anger, or fear.[35] The muscle weakness can be so severe that the person is almost paralyzed and might drop to the floor. The attack might be mistaken for an epileptic seizure. The episode can last for seconds or minutes, and then vanish.[36] Not all people afflicted with narcolepsy have all of these defining symptoms.

Narcolepsy can strike people of all ages; it usually peaks during adolescence. It affects about 0.05 percent of the population or one in 2,000 people. The first symptom is excessive daytime sleepiness, although hypnagogic hallucinations may be the first symptom, while cataplexy and sleep paralysis develop later.[37]

There is no cure, but some medications can control the symptoms. Modafinil (Provigil), a stimulant drug, is the first choice of treatment in helping afflicted people stay awake during the day. It is less abused than other stimulant medications. Some antidepressant medications help control episodes of cataplexy, sleep paralysis, and hypnagogic hallucinations. Lifestyle adjustments, such as avoiding heavy meals at bedtime and scheduling naps after meals may help to alleviate daytime sleepiness. Obviously, people with narcolepsy should not drive motor vehicles.[38]

The underlying causes of some sleep disorders or parasomnias are still unknown. Numerous medical, neurological, psychological, or psychiatric disorders cause sleep disturbances. Once treatments can be focused on the underlying problem, there is hope that the sleep disorder will be controlled. It appears that clonazepam, or related medications, are effective for most parasomnias.

Fatal Familial Insomnia

There is a known, but very, very rare and devastating disease called fatal familial insomnia (FFI). D.T. Max, in his book, *The Family Who Couldn't Sleep*, reveals the history of an Italian family whose many members were afflicted with this dread form of fatal insomnia.[39] The joint research into this disease and other diseases with similar brain pathology, by a couple of family members, physicians, and other scientists, finally led to some answers regarding the cause of the disease, and the resulting deaths of so many of the family members throughout the generations. It is mentioned here because the study of this disease has led researchers to discover the various brain structures responsible for sleep-awake states, and to better understand the various sleep disorders and causes of insomnia.

FFI is caused by a dominant autosomal mutation. This means that only one gene in an individual's DNA makeup is all that is necessary for this disease to be expressed. Therefore, there is a 50 percent probability that this mutant gene will be passed on to the offspring. If a child inherits this defective gene, the disease is not expressed until mid-life. This means that symptoms do not appear until the afflicted son or daughter reaches the mid-fifties. At the onset of the disease, some of the symptoms are sweating, constipation, menopause in women and impotency in men. Those afflicted soon begin to have trouble falling asleep. In about the next 15 months from the onset of symptoms, they fall into a state of exhaustion, then into a coma, and soon after die. It has never been understood why they actually died from this disease. The Italian family's inherited suffering has been known for at least the past two centuries.[40]

After years of investigating the cause and pathology of this disease, researchers discovered that it is caused by a malformed protein, known as a prion, which attacks the sleep center located at the base of the brain. There are only 40 known families worldwide that are afflicted with this condition. It was the study of this disease that led researchers to discover that the thalamus was the structure in the brain that controlled sleep.[41]

Researchers, through the years beginning about the 1960s, discovered brain pathology similar to that found in FFI in two other diseases: Creutzfeldt-

Jacob Disease (CJD) and Bovine Spongiform Encephalitis (BSE), more commonly known as "mad cow disease." Both of these diseases are caused by prions and lead to severe neurological symptoms and death. Prions are actually "infectious" mal-formed proteins that can cause disease in humans who have eaten infected cattle or other animals. Upon autopsy of infected individuals, under microscope examination of their brains, the thalamus and nearby structures were found to be badly damaged. Holes, plaque, and tangled proteins, similar to the pathology seen in the brains of Alzheimer's victims, were discovered.[42]

There is little hope of cure for FFI, but with today's ever expanding technology, a woman can be tested to see if she has this defective gene, when there is a known family history of FFI. She can then make a decision about not becoming pregnant, or not continuing a pregnancy, if that is her wish.

This story of FFI is a worst-case scenario. It is presented here to show what research has unfolded over the years. As stated earlier, sleep science is a relatively new field of research. Yet, there are already effective ways to treat most other forms of insomnia and sleep disorders. Ways to manage insomnia and sleep disorders are covered in more detail in Chapter 9. The next chapter details the many health effects and risks of sleep deprivation.

CHAPTER 8

The Consequences of Insomnia

Whatever the cause, for most people sleepless nights or disturbed sleep leaves them feeling tired or exhausted the next day. Mood is also affected. People usually feel irritable, down, or even depressed the day after a poor night's sleep. Chronic or long-term insomnia can lead to sleep deprivation with psychological and physical consequences. Not only are sufferers' general health at risk, but they are also at higher risk for injury or death from accidents in the workplace, on the road, in the sky, or on the sea.

Long-term insomnia can have profound effects on the person's quality of life, health, and economics. Chronic insomniacs have reported symptoms of depression, irritability, fatigue, decreased concentration, memory lapses, increased health problems, decreased productivity, and missed work days. The cost of treatment, including prescribed or over-the-counter medications, has ranged in the billions. According to Dr. David Neubauer, general education about sleep disorders is lacking and medical schools ignore, or devote minimal time, to sleep medicine.[1]

Of course, the effects of sleep deprivation vary according to its severity and individual differences on sleep needs and particular personality. As I have revealed in my own story, I feel tired, irritable, cranky, and even depressed if I don't sleep well. On the other hand, some people either deal with it better or function normally in spite of lost sleep; such is the case with Allen, as explained in his story. However, there are serious consequences in the long run when people build up significant sleep debt. Physical health can be compromised, leaving people more vulnerable to colds and infections. For example, it is well known that infectious mononucleosis ("mono") is more prevalent among college students than the general population. As discussed in Chapter 4, many in this young population are sleep deprived—not necessarily because of insomnia, but because of their lifestyle, heavy schedules, peer pressures, and individual choices. My grandson, who was recently graduated from a nearby university, is a typical example of the above pattern. He would go to sleep very late, either because he was out socializing with friends or studying. He has had several colds a year while attending the university.

As discussed in Chapter 2, one purpose of sleep (among others) is regulation of the body's immunologic processes. When our immune system is working up to par, specific white blood cells, macrophages (scavenger cells in our blood), and antibodies are ready to wage war against the constant pursuit of bacteria, viruses, and other microscopic critters ready to invade our bodies to cause all sorts of infections and ailments. A healthy immune system generally wins. However, a healthy immune system can be compromised if sleep is chronically deprived. When our immune system fails to do its job efficiently, we are more vulnerable to catching colds or other infectious diseases. A healthy immune system is also known to fight off certain cancers and other disease processes.

Results from one research study conducted on university students between the ages of 18 and 25 years have shown that those who get insufficient sleep (less than seven hours) on most nights had twice as many physician visits than those who slept more than seven hours of sleep a night. Other laboratory studies have shown similar results—that poor sleepers report poor health more often than good sleepers. Laboratory animal studies have also shown that sleep-deprived rats or mice lost weight, were unable to maintain normal body temperature, and died after a few weeks. Medical interns and residents, who are known to be sleep-deprived, are also plagued with colds, flu, and other infections.[2]

In a May 2010 news release from the Endocrine Society, Dr. Esther Donga, of the Leiden University Medical Center in the Netherlands and lead researcher of a study on the effects of insulin resistance on poor sleepers, claims that "just one sleepless night can cause insulin resistance, a component of type 2 diabetes." She further stated, "Our data indicate that insulin sensitivity is not fixed in healthy subjects, but depends on the duration of sleep in the preceding night." She added, "Our findings show a short night of sleep has more profound effects on metabolic regulation than previously appreciated." Dr. Donga claims, "Sleep duration has shortened considerably in western societies in the past decade and, simultaneously, there has been an increase in the prevalence of insulin resistance and type 2 diabetes."[3] The bottom line is that prolonged sleep deprivation can compromise our health in many ways.

Another purpose of good sleep, as explained in Chapter 2, is physical growth and tissue repair. Some laboratory studies have shown that sleep-deprived rats had impeded wound healing. Such studies, however, have been inconclusive. In other research studies conducted in the 1980s, rats were severely deprived of sleep. As soon as they fell asleep, they were stimulated with a turning disk and water to prevent them from sleeping. The researchers concluded that the rats died from exhaustion, since no other significant reason was found to cause the rats' deaths, upon autopsy.[4]

In his book, *Understanding Sleeplessness*, Dr. David Neubauer claims that long-term insomnia can have profound effects on health, quality of life, and economics. Research studies have shown that the consequences of long-term insomnia are, in addition to those mentioned above, decreased concentration, memory difficulty, less productivity at work, increased health problems leading to more missed work days, and overall greater health care costs, including the costs of medications.[5] Depending on how severe the sleep deprivation is, and individual variances, effects include general slowing down of mental processes, increased frustration level, and impaired motor and speech function. Furthermore, existing mental and physical ailments can become exacerbated.[6]

Sleep deprivation can lead to such physical health problems as heart disease, high blood pressure, kidney disease, and metabolic disorders. Results from a 2003 study involving 71,000 nurses showed that those who slept fewer than five hours in a 24-hour period were 45 percent more likely to develop heart disease when followed for ten years.[7] As discussed in Chapter 5, high blood pressure can result from severe sleep deficit, particularly in cases of obstructive sleep apnea. People suffering from OSA have a higher risk of heart attacks and strokes.

Earlier studies found relationships between weight gain in middle-aged women and poor sleep, but did not elucidate which came first. A later longitudinal study of 7,332 men and women of age 40 to 60 over the years 2002 to 2009 at the University of Helsinki, reported in the *Journal of Obesity*, showed that one-third of women with frequent sleep problems gained at least 11 pounds, whereas only one-fifth of those without problems gained weight. Men's sleep problems were not related to weight gain.[8] Hospital personnel who work long hours or swing shifts (rotating day, evening, and night shifts) are particularly vulnerable to sleep deprivation. As a nurse for many years, I have witnessed very sleepy medical interns and residents who have been on call for 24 hours or more. Sometimes they were fortunate enough to find some time to sleep during quiet nights, but other times, they just had to keep on going until their shift or "on-call" time was over. It is frightening to think what could go wrong when a sleep-deprived surgeon is operating. Things have gone wrong in the operating room, as well as in providing medical or nursing care. Many hospital medical personnel—physicians, anesthesiologists, nurses, and other health care workers—who work long hours and swing shifts are vulnerable to chronic sleep deprivation, and consequently, medical errors. Recalling my experience in Chapter 3 about working two nights per week as a hospital nurse in 1969, I did not fare very well and my kids suffered from that experience.

Reports in medical journals have revealed that medical residents have worked shifts that are as long as 30 hours twice a week. "One out of five first-year residents admits to making fatigue-related mistakes that resulted in injury to a patient." Some of these mistakes have resulted in the death of a patient.[9] This issue has been addressed for many years in healthcare settings. Hospital administrators work very hard to address these issues and continue to plan and implement safety strategies to prevent medical errors.

As stated several times, sleep deprivation can also lead to injury or death due to accidents in the workplace, on the road, on rails, in the air, or on the sea. For example, truck drivers can build up extensive sleep deprivation, particularly if they drive long distances for long hours into the night. Not only do they put themselves at great risk, but also place others in their wake at risk of sustaining severe injury or death. People who build up substantial sleep deficit are at risk for accidents sustained at work, particularly when handling dangerous equipment. The costs of work-related accidents have been in the billions. The Institute of Medicine (IOM) estimates that nearly 20 percent of all motor vehicle accidents are due to sleepy drivers.[10] Fatigue among 18- to 25-year-olds is also the number one cause of traffic accidents.[11] The IOM and the national scientific advisory group, "places medical costs of collective sleep debt at tens of billions of dollars. The loss in terms of work productivity is even higher." Add to this the loss of work, relationships, and enjoyment of life's pleasures.[12]

In 1988, the National Commission on Sleep Disorders reported that the cost of motor vehicle accidents caused by sleepiness was $37.9 billion that year. The cost of sleep-induced public transportation accidents was $720 million, and the cost of work-related accidents was $13.34 billion. The human costs of injury and death are even more alarming.[13]

These statistics bring to light the enormity of the problem. Major catastrophes have been related to sleep deprivation. The Exxon Valdez crash and subsequent oil spill in the Pacific Northwest was attributed to the captain's sleep debt. A recent metroliner crash in Washington, D.C. (in 2010), was also suspected to be caused by the engineer's sleepiness. Fatal airplane crashes have also been related to pilots' probable sleep deprivation.

A 2009 commuter jet en route from Newark, New Jersey, to Buffalo, New York, crashed, killing 49 people aboard and one on the ground. The

National Transportation Safety Board concluded that the pilot and copilot had had only sporadic amounts of sleep the day leading up to the crash. The cause of the accident was related to pilot fatigue.[14]

As mentioned above, truck drivers who are on the road for many hours, sometimes for 24 hours or more, build up a sizable amount of sleep debt. In the early 1990s, Dr. Dement pondered how many long-haul truck drivers suffered from obstructive sleep apnea. He conducted a study in which he questioned 602 truck drivers—ninety percent were male—and conducted overnight sleep recordings on 200 of them. The alarming results turned out to be that 70 percent were diagnosed with sleep apnea. He asked the drivers when they thought they should stop driving. "Eighty-two percent of the drivers replied that they would stop driving when they had a startle resulting from a head drop or when they saw something in the road that wasn't there (a hypnagogic hallucination)." Dement concluded that "both of these events signal that they had already fallen asleep at the wheel."[15] I never have felt comfortable sharing the road with big tractor-trailer trucks. After reading this story, I am more leery than ever.

It is obvious that sleep deprivation, whatever the cause, has significant effects on personal health and safety, safety of others, economics, social and emotional well-being, and physical and cognitive functioning. Sleep specialists contend that not enough is being done to understand the root causes of insomnia and that it is generally undertreated. According to D. T. Max, "...little is being done to understand the root causes of insomnia. Most medical school students get no more than four hours of training on sleep disorders; some get none. Family doctors' health questionnaires often don't even ask about sleep."[16] Although research continues to discover the complexities of sleep—why it is so important for health, growth, tissue repair and restoration, and what the consequences of sleep debt are—there is still so much to learn.

There is help for sufferers of insomnia and other sleep disorders. The important thing is to recognize symptoms (what your body is trying to tell you), how insomnia and other sleep disorders affect you, and that there are remedies for many sleep problems. The next chapter explores the many options of treatments that relieve and manage sleep problems and specific sleep disorders.

CHAPTER 9

Management of Insomnia

If you have established that you have insomnia and are not happy about the way you feel during your waking hours, what are you going to do about it? As stated several times, insomnia is usually a symptom of some other problems—certain stresses, unknown causes (primary insomnia), medical conditions that need diagnosis, depression or other psychological disorders, or a specific underlying sleep disorder, such as obstructive sleep apnea, restless leg syndrome, or a parasomnia that disrupts normal sleep. Obviously, the underlying problem should be treated first if at all possible, as suggested in Chapters 5 and 7. Many underlying causes of insomnia, specific sleep disorders, and parasomnias can be treated by tried and effective methods. Once the underlying problem is resolved, then the sleep problem will (hopefully) likewise be resolved. However, identification or diagnosis of underlying problem(s) is not always possible. Such primary insomnias can be complex and disturbing for many people.

So, if you are troubled with some form of insomnia—you are unable to fall asleep or maintain a restful night's sleep, and feel exhausted the next day—the first thing you should do is seek medical care. You should relate all of your symptoms and a complete profile of your history of sleep disturbance symptoms to your health care provider. Hopefully the basic problem can be identified. Evaluation at a sleep lab might be indicated.

However, for people who have true (primary or idiosyncratic) insomnias, treatment becomes a little more complicated. Primary insomnia is sometimes referred to as "psycho-physiological insomnia." There can be acute or temporary causes of insomnia related to physical illness, pain, psychological factors, such as depression and stress. When these issues can be identified and resolved, in many cases the insomnia is also resolved, but not always. Often, the stressors in our lives can be as minor as worrying about getting up in time for work, or as major as a crisis happening at work or at home. Whatever the cause or situation in your life and the character of your sleep problems, there are options. The first things you should become aware of are your usual habits and routines in preparing for sleep.

Sleep Hygiene

According to Dr. Dement, "The simple goal of good sleep hygiene is to do everything possible to foster good sleep at night."[1] Good sleep hygiene is a universal set of rules, such as avoiding caffeinated beverages and alcohol at bedtime, not exercising in the evening (it is helpful to exercise earlier in the day), and keeping a regular schedule of going to sleep at the same time every night and arising at the same time every morning. Caffeine is a stimulant drug that has a long half-life, meaning it can still be in your system for up to six hours or so. Alcohol has an initial sedating effect, but after a couple of hours, it has a rebound stimulating effect. It also blocks the anti-diuretic hormone, secreted by the pituitary gland. Consequently, you have to urinate frequently when you are trying to sleep. Drink plenty of water during the day. Actually, if you are dehydrated, you have to urinate more frequently because your urine becomes more acidic, which is irritating to the urinary bladder.

Avoid daytime naps if possible. Your bedroom should be dark and well-ventilated when you are ready to go to sleep. It is best to use your bed only for sleep and sex. Avoid reading a stimulating book, watching an action-packed movie on television, or engaging in other stimulating activities. Also avoid using a computer in your bedroom. It is important to go to sleep when sleepy and sleep in a dark room. This set of rules has been included in just about every book I've read on insomnia.

Keep in mind that such "rules" don't work for everyone. There are differences in our chemistry and disposition that makes us all unique in many aspects of our lives. I, for one, usually read in bed, which makes me sleepy (if it's not a page-turning mystery). I am so tired at the end of the day I just need to get horizontal—in bed (usually by nine). I do try to avoid reading suspenseful or action-packed mysteries. However, I can't seem to fall asleep without reading something in bed.

People, in general, are creatures of habit. We tend to follow certain routines that we are comfortable with and do not want to change. If our ritual routine in preparing for sleep works, we should stick with it. According to a recent study on older adults, results showed that those people who kept regular routines throughout the day experienced better sleep than those who did not keep such regular routines. According to Michael J. Breus, PhD (the "Sleep Doctor"), "The body loves routines. Each one of us maintains a circadian rhythm that dictates our sleep-wake cycles. This rhythm clocks our biological days and takes cues from light and darkness."[2]

Medications

Medical treatment is aimed at relieving symptoms, so when other underlying causes are ruled out, sleeping pills are generally prescribed. According to D.T. Max, "Fifty to 75 million Americans, roughly a fifth of the population, complain about problems sleeping. Fifty-six million prescriptions for sleeping pills were written in 2008, up 54 percent over the previous four years."[3] (Apparently, Max's last sentence means that annual prescriptions for sleeping pills rose 54 percent between 2003 and the end of 2008.) Many people with whom I've talked have revealed that they have insomnia, but refuse to take sleeping pills. Sleeping pills, medically referred to as hypnotic medications, are effective for most people. However, there are downsides to taking some formulations of sleeping pills; many are physically and psychologically addictive and have other side effects. Newer sleep medications have fewer side effects and are not physically addicting.

Most hypnotics act upon the limbic system of the brain. This is an area in the mid-brain (near the base of the brain) that is comprised of several structures, such as the thalamus, hypothalamus, and other centers that govern circadian rhythms and regulate memory formation during REM sleep. These centers also regulate human emotions and behavior, and other processes. Chemicals in this area of the brain, called neurotransmitters, mediate these various processes and functions. Neurotransmitters, also referred to as neurochemicals, are released between nerve endings, to carry out specific functions. The effect the neurotransmitters have on the nerves they innervate is either stimulating or inhibiting. This means that a neurotransmitter either causes a specific reaction or inhibits it.

An important inhibitory neurotransmitter, gamma-aminobutyric acid (GABA), regulates sleep, alertness, and emotions. This neurotransmitter renders the nerve cells less reactive to stimuli. Many hypnotic medications (sleeping pills) act upon this system. A family of hypnotic and sedative drugs, the benzodiazepines, stimulates the action of GABA. Since GABA is inhibitory, this area of the brain is not stimulated, but instead is slowed down. Then, the overall effect is sedation. Dysfunction of GABA might be linked to certain anxiety disorders.[4]

The many hypnotic drugs in the family of benzodiazepines (having similar chemical structure) fall into groups of short-acting, intermediate-acting, and long-acting medications. The short-acting group of drugs is absorbed rapidly into the circulation and travels to our brains. The effect lasts about two to five hours. The intermediate group is also absorbed fairly rapidly, but lasts five to twenty hours. An example is temazepam (Restoril). (Trade names of drugs are capitalized and are in parentheses.) Long-acting drugs, such as diazepam (Valium) and flurazepam (Dalmane), are absorbed quickly, but last about two to four days. This explains why long-acting benzodiazepines hang on during the daytime and yield hangover symptoms.[5]

Long-acting benzodiazepines are better for treating anxiety than for treating insomnia, because their effects last well beyond the night. One of the earliest of this group is chlordiazepoxide (Librium), which came on the market in the 1960s. It is an effective drug used in treating depression. Valium soon followed, and became one of the most popular drugs for treating both anxiety and insomnia. Valium is effective in treating anxiety and seizure disorders, muscle spasm, and relieving symptoms of alcohol withdrawal. However, Valium is a poor drug of choice in treating insomnia because of its long half-life, and also because it has several central nervous system side effects. These side effects include depression, physical and psychological addiction, dizziness, daytime drowsiness, slowing down of thought processes, confusion, rebound insomnia, and more. Of course, as with any medication, side effects vary in degree according to individual differences. As a matter of fact, all of the benzodiazepines have these side effects, which vary in kind and severity among the many drugs in this family.

Another down side of many hypnotic sleeping pills is that the sleep they induce is not a natural one. The effects on sleep are a decrease in the amount of time spent in deep sleep and increase in the time spent in "twilight sleep" (stages 1 and 2). Hypnotic drugs also cause a delay in REM sleep as well as the overall time spent in this stage. Consequently, there are longer amounts of time spent in REM sleep during the last couple of cycles of the night, close to morning. Dreams occurring in the early morning are frequently disturbing.[6] However, this is not the case with the latest group of hypnotic medications.

More recent hypnotics are the "Z" drugs (in the family of imidazopyridines). These include zopiclone (Imovane), eszopiolone (Lunesta), zaleplon (Sonata), and zolpidem (Ambien). Hypnotics in this group are short-acting and have short half-lives. This means that these hypnotics are absorbed and eliminated quickly. They also produce a more normal sleep pattern than the older group of sleep aids. These hypnotics shorten the time it takes to fall asleep, improve quality of sleep, and reduce the number of awakenings. Also, these newer products seem to have fewer side effects than the older hypnotic drugs, although they still have some similar, but milder, side effects such as daytime drowsiness, dizziness, headaches, and dryness of the mouth.[7] I (Phyllis) take the lowest dose of zolpidem (Ambien) when I have difficulty falling asleep, but not on a regular basis. It has been very effective for me. The only side effect I experience is dry mouth. Just knowing I can take something to help me fall asleep when I am unable to do so eases my anxiety over not being able to fall asleep.

Most of the earlier sleeping pills were physically or psychologically addictive to some extent. The most troublesome ill effects of taking the older hypnotic drugs occur when the individual stops taking them. These are the "withdrawal" effects (most prominent in the barbiturates and benzodiazepines) that are similar to the withdrawal symptoms of alcoholics. These symptoms range from feelings of anxiety, depression, and confusion, loss of appetite, tremors, and sweating. Some people may even experience psychotic episodes.[8] Not all of these symptoms occur in all people withdrawing from taking these drugs or in the same degree of severity. The newer "Z" group of hypnotics is not addicting, so people using these sleep aids do not suffer withdrawal symptoms when stopping the medication.

Most of the earliest sleeping pills that I can remember, back in the 1950s, were a family of drugs called barbiturates. Common sleeping pills in this category are Nembutal, Seconal, and Phenobarbital. These drugs cause general depression of the brain and are highly addictive. Side effects include tolerance (decreasing effect, requiring higher doses over time), physical and psychological dependence, hangover, drowsiness, nausea, depression, blood disorders, and other medical problems. Withdrawal symptoms occur when the medication is stopped. Barbiturates are rarely used today for insomnia, but some are used as anesthesia for surgical procedures. Phenobarbital is used therapeutically to control seizures resulting from epilepsy or other neurological pathology. Other hypnotics that have been tried through the years are chloral hydrate and some anti-depressant drugs.

Severe or unexpected side effects of any medication are referred to as "adverse effects." Some people have unexpected serious effects, such as allergic reactions or blood disorders. When taking sleeping pills, it is very important *not* to take other central nervous system depressant medications or alcohol at the same time. These drugs potentiate the effects of the sleep medication. The side effects mentioned above can severely worsen and even be fatal in some individuals. Most medications are metabolized in the liver and excreted from the kidneys. People who have diseases in these organs are more susceptible to the side effects and adverse effects of these medications. Overdoses of any sedative or hypnotic drug can cause coma and death.

Older people are more vulnerable to the side effects of many medications, particularly hypnotic and other sedative drugs. They may respond to
hypnotics by becoming over-sedated, confused, dizzy, and unsteady with
risk of falling. Smaller doses should be prescribed to older adults.[9] It is also
important to stress that they should *not* take other sedative-type medications
or drink alcohol beverages, while taking sleeping pills.

There are sometimes conflicting attitudes in the use of sleeping pills for
treating insomnia among health professionals and people who are troubled
with insomnia. Among the books I've used as resources for writing this book,
some authors paint a very negative picture, while others have more positive
views. Dr. Dement, who has been a sleep specialist for decades, concluded
that in a recent survey of students in his "Sleep and Dreams" course, 94 percent of the students strongly believed that sleeping pills are addicting. He
points out that there is no evidence that newer prescription sleep medications
are addicting. In 1983, a panel of sleep experts at a conference sponsored by
the National Institutes of Health all agreed that "safe and effective sleep
medication is the treatment of choice for transient insomnia." Dement contends that, in addition to the misinformed public, many physicians still believe
that sleeping pills are addicting and have serious side-effects.[10]

In the long run, hypnotic medications are effective in helping to improve
sleep time and quality, as well as improving general health, ability to function
during the day, and the quality of life. Aside from using hypnotics, there are
other methods (described later in this chapter) that have been shown to be
effective in treating insomnia.

Ten hypnotic medications have been approved by the U.S. Food and Drug
Administration (FDA). However, only two of them, eszopiclone (Lunesta)
and zolpidem (Ambien) have been evaluated for efficacy in people with co-
morbidities (co-existing medical or psychiatric conditions). Research has
shown that a combination of hypnotic medications and cognitive behavioral
therapies are effective in treating people who have insomnia and co-existing
chronic disorders. Dr. David Neubauer has emphasized that clinicians should
"customize treatments for patients with co-morbid insomnia based upon co-
existing medical and psychiatric disorders, age, medical history, current medications, and lifestyle issues."[11]

In addition to the sedative and hypnotic effects, sleeping medications
may also have a psychological effect. It does so for me because knowing I
have a back-up plan, I'm not as anxious over not being able to fall asleep.
Sleeping pills are not for everyone who has sleep issues and are not the final
solution to treating insomnia. It is best to take them for a limited period of
time and to take the lowest dose possible at the start of a treatment regimen.

The hypnotic drugs discussed so far can only be obtained by prescription from a licensed health care provider with prescriptive authority, such as a physician or nurse practitioner. There are sleep remedies that can be purchased over-the-counter (OTC) that are regulated and regarded as safe if taken as directed on the container label. OTC sleep aids mostly contain antihistamines, such as Benadryl. The main purpose of this group of drugs is to treat allergies, acute allergic reactions and nasal congestion; some are also effective in treating nausea and vomiting, such as in seasickness. Actually it is one of the side effects of this group of antihistamines, that of sedation, that acts as a hypnotic.

As with any medication, non-prescription (OTC) medications also have side effects similar to those of prescription hypnotics. Some of these side effects include next day drowsiness, poor coordination, blurred vision, dry mouth, and headaches. Antihistamines can also have the opposite effect of sedation and cause agitation and sleeplessness.[12] People with health conditions and older people should not take any OTC sleep-inducing medications without first consulting a healthcare provider. As established with prescription sleep medications, OTC hypnotic medications might work for some people, but have no effect for others.

Another sleep remedy for temporary insomnia is melatonin. As explained in Chapter 2, melatonin is a natural hormone synthesized in the pineal gland that is secreted in response to darkness. It can help shift the natural circadian rhythm in some circumstances. Melatonin is approved by the federal Food and Drug Administration (FDA) as a food additive. In small doses, it might help some people who have trouble falling asleep, especially when it is related to jet lag or shift work. One of the side effects of melatonin is constriction of blood vessels, so people who have cardiovascular disease could be at risk.[13]

Herbal Remedies

Herbal remedies are another option for some people who are troubled by insomnia, yet don't like the idea of taking prescription or OTC medications. The identification of the sleep potential properties of various herbal remedies has largely been by trial and error through the ages. Of course, the basis of many commonly used medications has been identified through trial and error in the earliest of times. The difference is that prescription and OTC medications have been scientifically investigated as safe and then approved and regulated by the federal Food and Drug Administration (FDA). Herbal and other home remedy products have not gone through this process, and are, therefore, unregulated. Safety could be a concern, but general consensus of effectiveness and safety by those taking these preparations without unto-ward side effects probably renders them safe. They are, after all, natural herbs.

Some of the herbal preparations are valerian, chamomile tea, lemon balm tea, and verbena. People who have used these preparations have claimed that their sleep improved. Another natural hypnotic is tryptophan, which is actually an amino acid (one of the many molecules that make up proteins that are essential to the human diet). Dairy products are rich in tryptophan. Clinical trials have shown that tryptophan is effective; it shortens the time in falling asleep and decreases the number of awakenings during the night. It doesn't work for everyone, but was shown to be effective for 60 to 70 percent of those taking it.[14] Since milk is high in tryptophan, it might help to drink a glass of milk prior to retiring for the night. Phyllis does this on occasion after zapping it in the microwave for a minute. It does, at times, help her fall asleep faster. Sleeping pills—whether prescription, OTC, or herbal—might not be the choice for all insomniacs. There are other ways to promote better sleep.

Alternative Methods

There are several alternative methods that are effective in promoting sleep for some people. According to Dr. Dement, alternative methods have been tried, but not truly tested. Some of these methods include hypnosis, yoga, biofeedback, massage, and herbal remedies. Hypnosis demands pres-ence of a hypnotist, so how would this work? Would you invite the hypnotist into your bedroom at night? I think not. The hypnosis occurs in the doctor's office and lasts for some period of time. Also, a hypnotic trance is not the same as natural sleep. Self-hypnosis, meditation, and yoga have similar com-ponents of progressive relaxation, which is slow, rhythmic breathing while tensing and then relaxing all muscle groups progressively from head to toe.[15] I would think that these methods would be more feasible than hypnosis.

I taught childbirth preparation classes for many years. I taught progres-sive relaxation techniques, which couples practiced, along with other relax-ation exercises. Many a couple fell asleep during these practice sessions. However, on many occasions when I had trouble sleeping, I tried to practice what I preached. It didn't work for me. My own anxiety and worry over my perceived inability to sleep counteracted the effects of progressive relaxation. What can I say? Other relaxation techniques, such as listening to soft, lullaby music and massage (by your partner) works for some people, and has helped me. Acupuncture is another possible method for relieving symptoms of insomnia.

Psychotherapy

Psychotherapy plays an important role in the treatment of insomnia symptoms, as well as in dealing with people's issues related to life stressors. Psychotherapeutic methods are based on people's personal stories about their experiences with insomnia. These methods are aimed at treating people with chronic insomnia without known underlying medical or sleep disorder pathology. The therapeutic approach involves initial evaluation of the individual's story about when and how the symptoms began and how they affected the individual's life.[16]

A global model for evaluating these symptoms considers three components of the individual's story: predisposing, precipitating, and perpetuating factors. *Predisposing* factors include personality vulnerabilities, circadian rhythm tendency, and lifestyle. *Precipitating* factors might be situational crises (grief/loss), medical or surgical illness, substance use, schedule changes, or other life events that may have initiated symptoms of insomnia. *Perpetuating* factors are new situations that sustain the symptoms, such as daytime napping, alcohol consumption at bedtime, and conditioned hyperarousal states.[17] The type of therapy employed is directed at understanding and then correcting the underlying problems derived from the individual's story, as well as common symptoms shared by others. The three therapeutic approaches, described by Dr. David Neubauer in his book *Understanding Sleeplessness*, are sleep restriction, stimulus control, and cognitive behavioral therapy.

Sleep restriction is a method of therapy used for people who spend long hours in bed, who are unable to sleep or who fail to experience sufficient, refreshing sleep. Therefore, the underlying basis of excessive wakefulness is perpetuated. The strategy is then to limit the time spent awake in bed by delaying the person's usual bedtime. At the start of therapy, there is some sleep deficit, but as sleep improves, the bedtime is moved to an earlier time.[18]

Stimulus control is based on the theory that the person's anxiety is related to bedtime rituals associated with preparing for sleep. This anxiety then creates a conditioned hyperarousal state. This negative response is perpetuated and becomes a vicious cycle. The goal of therapy is to decondition the response by eliminating the factors that reinforce the hyperarousal state. To do this, the person is instructed to delay bedtime until he or she is sleepy and, if still awake after ten minutes, to get out of bed and try again later. The person should also refrain from taking daytime naps. There might be temporary sleep deprivation with this method, but it is soon outweighed by the beneficial effects of therapy.[19]

Cognitive-behavioral therapy (CBT) is based on the principle that a person's feelings and behaviors are derived from his or her experiences in life. Treatment is directed toward identifying and correcting dysfunctional beliefs and attitudes, irrational fears, and unrealistic expectations. Once they have difficulty sleeping, their fear exacerbates the problem. Neubauer states, "There seems to be a self-fulfilling prophecy in the anticipation of sleepless misery." Therapy focuses on educating the patient about healthy sleep practices, and correcting and redirecting misconceptions and cognitive distortions.[20] The therapist teaches the person to think about his or her problem as manageable and solvable, and to practice good sleep hygiene. Depending on the basis of the insomnia problem, CBT is not effective for all insomniacs, but is offered as a potential cure for many.[21]

In addition to treating insomnia, cognitive-behavioral therapy has also been used to treat depression, anxiety, chronic pain, and addiction. Experts estimate that 70 to 80 percent of people with chronic insomnia can benefit from this type of treatment. CBT strives to change the unhelpful attitudes and beliefs that cause anxiety and arouse the body, all of which make sleep difficult. The therapist helps the person restructure negative, disturbing thoughts.[22]

There is research evidence that psychological and behavioral therapies are effective for people who have primary insomnia. A systematic review of 37 behavioral treatment studies, conducted between 1998 and 2004, found that "psychological and behavioral therapies produced reliable changes in several sleep parameters in individuals with either primary insomnia or insomnia associated with medical and psychiatric disorders." The research review also showed that improvements in sleep were sustained over time.[23]

A Final Word

If none of the above methods for managing insomnia works for you or doesn't seem to be what you would choose to use, there is one other option. As my husband has said to me many times, "If you are miserable, you might as well enjoy it." I am not advocating this message, but Sondra Kornblatt, in her book *Restful Insomnia*, offers some helpful advice. She advocates good sleep hygiene, as discussed repeatedly in her book and in all the books I've read relating to insomnia. She also suggests acupuncture. However, when nothing seems to work, she says, "The Restful Insomnia approach is avant-garde...."[24] It is reframing how you look at insomnia—changing how you view insomnia, which is not a bad thing. It is also looking at it from a new perspective. Kornblatt provides many examples and analogies to the process.

Some tips she offers are reading (material that is not upsetting), darkness and evening rituals, and not worrying about falling asleep.[25]

At the time of this writing, I have had several nights when I just couldn't fall asleep without the help of my Ambien. I have been reading Kornblatt's book in the evenings. One night (or early morning), my husband got in very late from being out of town for the day. I awoke at 4:15 in the morning, when he was just getting in. So, of course, I was then wide awake, but too tired to get up. However, I struggled into the kitchen, drank a cup of warm milk, and got back in bed. I didn't worry about falling back to sleep, so I just lay there and let my thoughts drift. Lo and behold, I fell back to sleep. Bottom line is, I think Kornblatt has some good ideas.

There is hope for the many insomniacs out there. There are many treatment options, be it medication, herbal remedies, alternative methods, or psychotherapy. The main objective is to seek medical evaluation for any possible underlying causes, which should first be treated or managed. If primary insomnia is the diagnosis, the person should be educated in regards to the many available options, as well as some side effects of medications. Then, the person (maybe you) will be enabled to make an informed choice about which option is best.

CHAPTER 10

Composite Analyses of Symptoms, Causes, Effects, and Remedies for Insomnia

Preamble

Phyllis, the nurse educator and originator of this book, searched the medical and popular book and article literature and wrote all of the difficult chapters that provide the reader with a capsule view and the terminology of the physiological and medical aspects of insomnia. She is my energizer bunny and does everything "yesterday." After I (Allen) had contributed only to the easier, less technical Chapters 3 and 6, she prevailed upon me to write this chapter to earn my place on the front cover. More than earning my place on the front cover, I want to stay out of the doghouse.

About This Chapter

This chapter will assemble the main facts about insomnia from the literature and questionnaires for reference in the following categories:

1. Symptoms and sleep measurements characterizing insomnia
2. Causes of sleep problems
3. Effects of sleep loss
4. Remedies for improving sleep and their associated effectiveness

In presenting and discussing this composite information, two tables have been constructed from information in the questionnaires for (2) causes and

(4) remedies. No table will be used for the symptoms of category (1) above, because all of the information about symptoms has been extracted in Chapter 6 following the narratives. The information has been presented in Chapter 6 using the ten modified symptom categories of Neubauer[1] in Chapter 6.

The reasons for having modified the symptom categories of Neubauer may be summarized as follows. First of all, the reasons are related to the fact that it is likely that only the more severe cases of insomnia, those that cannot be "lived with," are likely to seek medical help. This fact is evident in our respondent sample. Persons coming to Neubauer's sleep center have necessarily been categorized according to symptoms as they are presented to a healthcare provider. Persons presenting themselves to a healthcare provider usually come in with symptoms that are severe, and cause severe suffering. Therefore, as presented by Neubauer, the ten symptoms listed in his book are each listed as always bothersome, or totally present. Therefore, for use in this book on living with insomnia, modifications of Neubauer's categories were necessary to include in our narratives persons who had significant suffering and adverse effects some of the time, but who were able on their own to find ways to live with their occasional or frequent sleep problems and carry on with a productive and satisfying life. In this way, with the ten modified categories, all of the important information on symptoms has been extracted from the questionnaires in Chapter 6, and presented in that chapter in several ways.

Section 3, effects of insomnia, will not require a table, because the effects are commonly experienced by almost everyone who loses a night's sleep once in awhile, in addition to insomniacs. These effects include tiredness during daytime activities that prevent productivity during work or enjoyment during recreation. These effects are well known and discussions of these effects in previous chapters suffice for this book and will be easily remembered.

Tables are presented in the sections below on causes of sleeplessness and remedies to improve sleep, because more information can be extracted from our sample of narratives by the use of tables that give an overview of the information and allow further observations and conclusions. Causes of sleep loss deserve more examination because a focus on elimination of these causes can improve conditions for good sleep. In the same way, the explicit examination of remedies used by our respondents deserves more emphasis for providing help to those suffering from insomnia. At the beginning of each table, symbols have been defined that appear in the boxes within the table for each respondent and each sleep issue deemed important in analyzing the data. In this way, we have obtained tables from which we can observe and present to the reader the more important findings from our sample of respondents that are likely to help the reader. Simple use of X, O, or blanks would not capture all of the information needed for optimum analyses. However, we have carefully restricted the number of symbols and columns to include only the more valuable information, and to avoid too much complexity and difficulty for those who might seek their own overview of the information in the samples. We have tried to balance complexity with lucidity.

Because the tables have been followed by paragraphs presenting the important observations that can be drawn from them, it is not necessary for the busy reader to examine and understand the tables in detail. Some persons more interested in research or details of the data sample might want to spend more time examining the tables than others. Thus, it is noted here that the tables themselves may be just skimmed over or ignored by those readers who just want to obtain facts and findings related to improvements in sleep experience. However, reference back to numbered narratives in the tables will allow the reader to find narratives that match most closely to his own causes or remedies, in order to be able to go back to Chapter 6 and read just the narratives that pertain to his own sleep patterns and problems.

Symptoms and Sleep Measurements Characterizing Insomnia

Symptoms

As we have learned from previous chapters, there are many symptoms of insufficient sleep. If symptoms are defined as those we can observe from a person's behavior, or obtain from an oral medical history of complaints, then there are other possible characteristics of insomnia that might be uncovered from the kinds of brain wave studies discussed early. As described above, Neubauer[2] condensed the symptoms reported by persons concerned with sleep loss into ten complaints. Those complaints are repeated again from Chapter 6, for ease of reference in the discussions of this chapter:

1. I take too long to fall asleep at night.
2. I awaken through the night, like every hour.
3. I never get deep sleep anymore, and am always in a twilight state.
4. I have not slept in months.
5. I wake up too early and cannot get back to sleep.
6. I cannot shut off my mind at night.

7. I drag myself out of bed in the morning because my sleep is so bad.
8. I never feel rested.
9. I am fatigued all day.
10. I could not nap even if my life depended upon it.

As we have used these ten complaint symptoms in Chapter 6, the first six are the problems with sleeping, and the next four are the effects felt the next day upon awakening. As we have indicated in Chapter 6 and above, we needed to consider the frequency and severity of these symptoms in placing our questionnaire respondents into the categories of Chapter 6. As indicated in Chapter 5, it is rare that anyone has insomnia every night for months or years. Without considering frequency and severity, it was difficult to classify men and women into the three categories in Chapter 6 of having no serious sleep problems; having significant sleep problems that the person would like to alleviate, but is living with; or having sleep problems that deeply concern the individual and seriously affect his/her life.

In classifying persons as not having insomnia, living with insomnia, or having debilitating insomnia, we made use of another of Neubauer's insights, obtained after he described the variety and inconsistency of ways other authors defined insomnia. We adopted, and repeat again for coherence in this chapter, Neubauer's simple definition of insomnia:

"Fundamentally, 'I have insomnia' means (1) 'I can't sleep' and (2) 'I'm suffering.'"[3]

The degree to which the last four complaints (7 to 10 of Neubauer) represented serious debilitation in work accomplishments or lifestyles ("suffering") required judgments in order to place persons into the six categories (three for each sex) in Chapter 6.

So, in estimating the fraction of persons in our limited sample population that could be defined as having insomnia, we counted all of those in the third category and half of those in the second category to allow for our uncertainties in judgment. This results in the fact that almost half of our sample is interpreted as having insomnia, and this includes more women than men. This turns out to be consistent with the range of estimates in Chapter 1 of the percentages of persons who have insomnia, and the findings that more women suffer from insomnia than men. This result from our sample is particularly consistent with a report that about one-third to one-half of adults in the United States and other Western nations have experienced insomnia within the past year.[4]

Therefore, reader, if you think that you have insomnia, you are in good company.

Sleep center measurements: As stated in the first paragraph of this section, there are instrument measurements and observations, in addition to the symptoms observed or recorded by the individual or his health provider that can assist in cases of insomnia that are more difficult to diagnose and treat using symptoms only obtained in the physician's office or at home. The reader who cannot obtain relief from serious effects of insomnia from diagnosis of the usual symptoms alone should seek help at a sleep center, one that is well equipped with up-to-date technology and equipment and staffed by certified health care providers and physicians. Physicians associated with such sleep centers can then use both the subjective and objective symptoms of the patient, in addition to the center's instrument scans and traces, to better diagnose and treat the more serious cases of insomnia using the identifiable underlying causes.

The second chapter, which discusses mainly normal sleep patterns, has described the various instrument determinations used in sleep centers. Normal sleep patterns must be summarized here before abnormal patterns can be understood. As reviewed in Chapter 2, the mysteries of sleep and their disorders have been revealed since about the 1950s in experiments with instruments attached to, or adjacent to, the human body. Electrodes placed on the head with conducting leads to instruments that record electrical signals in various parts of the brain are known as electroencephalograms (EEG). These EEGs have identified, and can reveal in a patient, the durations of the various stages of sleep described in Chapter 2. Other sleep tests that can now be performed in a sleep center are the electromyogram (EMG), which records electrical activity in skeletal muscles and can detect muscle twitching during sleep; the electro-oculogram (EOG), which can characterize the rapid eye movement (REM) stages of sleep; and the electrocardiogram (ECG), which records the heart's electrical activity to indicate heart rate and normal function. Most everyone has seen the continuous tracings of an ECG in a hospital or doctor's office.

Also used to evaluate sleep patterns are monitors of audiovisual monitoring, and a multiple sleep latency test (MSLT) that determines sleep delays or onsets. Together, all of these tests conducted in a sleep lab are denoted as polysonogram diagnostics.

Using such diagnostics, the physician can obtain relationships between electrical signals in various areas of the brain and relate them to physiological responses detected by the other polysonogram determinations, and to symptoms. The measurements characterize the patient's relative amounts and durations of stages during sleep, and the patient's brain signals while awake, as the patient remains in the sleep center.

These changes in sleep stages and their relationships to other physiological or pathological conditions cannot be observed or interpreted from symptoms alone as provided in taking a medical history, and they can be important in uncovering underlying pathology related to the more serious sleep problems. The underlying pathology might itself require urgent treatment, which in turn then improves sleep. The amounts of sleep in the various stages is important to general health as well as to the restitution of energy for daily activities.

The sleep stages discussed in more detail in Chapter 2 are summarized here, with reference to the picture of graphs in Chapter 2.

When a person is awake, the ECG pattern shows a high-frequency, low-amplitude pattern, these are called "beta waves." As a person becomes relaxed and calm, just before falling asleep, the beta waves change to a slower-frequency and higher-amplitude pattern called "alpha waves." When the person enters the first stage of sleep, the alpha waves change to waves of an even slower frequency and higher amplitude, which are called "theta waves." This stage 1 of sleep can last about five or ten minutes and is characterized by complete relaxation, although the person can be easily awakened from this stage. On entering stage 2, the waves become even lower in frequency but are mixed with sporadic bursts of more frequent waves called spindles and K complexes. In stage 2, which lasts about five to ten minutes, the person is in a moderately light sleep. When stage 2 transitions to stage 3, the person descends into a deep sleep, with another pattern of low-frequency and high-amplitude brain waves that are designated as "delta waves." When these delta waves of stage 3 reach their slowest frequency and highest amplitude, the person has transitioned into the deepest stage of sleep, stage 4. This deepest stage of sleep is accompanied by a decreased heart rate, a slower and regular respiratory rate, and a lower body temperature. It is difficult to arouse a person in this stage 4 of sleep. Stage 4 lasts about 45 minutes in normal sleep, returning to stage 3 for about another ten minutes. Because wave patterns are similar for stages 3 and 4, some experts lump them together. After stage 4, the person drifts back to REM sleep, and the cycle can repeat itself, perhaps every 90 minutes or so in normal sleep, through the night if the person remains asleep.

The discovery of REM sleep, how it is related to signals in parts of the brain, and its relationship to dreams that sometimes can be remembered upon wakening, are described in Chapter 2. Images of the brain during REM sleep show an increased flow of blood to the brain. Dreams during REM sleep can sometimes be remembered after waking naturally, and were easily remembered when a subject was awakened during REM sleep in human experiments. However, it is now believed that these dreams are random and do not necessarily have meaningful interpretations. Nevertheless, current scientific evidence indicates that, during REM sleep, important conceptual learning, memory consolidation, and other improvements related to cognitive function take place.

In contrast, the deeper stages of sleep, 3 and 4, are the stages during which the body achieves its needed rest, and during which growth hormones are released that in early life promote physical growth and in adulthood are still needed for tissue repair and replacement.

The increase in sleep problems with age can be attributed to decreases in both REM sleep and deep sleep that seems to be correlated with increasing age past middle age. However, for reasons given in Chapter 2, we do not subscribe to interpretations that there is necessarily a decrease in REM sleep with age for all individuals, nor that any decrease in REM sleep is a cause for decreased memory capacity.

In any event, we hope that now the reader can better understand the importance of seeking sleep center studies and related medical evaluations in case of serious insomnia, in which remedies based on observable symptoms are insufficient.

However, if you suspect that you or your healthcare provider might help improve your sleep experiences just from examining your symptoms and lifestyle goals, read on to the rest of this chapter and the conclusions for a review of external causes and lifestyles that can be changed to improve sleep; how those external causes feed into and affect the brain and hormone balances that influence sleep-wake cycles; how sleep loss affects many aspects of your life and health; and how treatments and remedies can feed back to improve your sleep experience, health, and lifestyle.

Causes of Sleep Problems

For convenience in reviewing the causes of sleep problems or insomnia, this section is divided into (1) *external causes and conditions under the person's control* (e.g., lifestyles, pre-bedtime habits, poor sleep hygiene); and (2) *internal causes* (e.g., physical or psychological disorders not controlled by the individual and possibly needing medical diagnosis and treatment, including some parasomnias that accompany sleep and cause insomnia); and (3) *intrinsic causes initiated by (1) and (2)* (e.g. signals to the brain, initiated by the senses, and the resulting secretion of hormones that affect the sleep-wake cycle).

(1) EXTERNAL CAUSES AND CONDITIONS
UNDER THE PERSON'S CONTROL

Some of the most prevalent external causes are those of bad sleep hygiene, some of which are portrayed in the cartoon on page 153. The cartoon shows the worst of these: staying up late and not allowing enough time for sleep before the next day's obligations; the eyes focused on intense, glaring images and loud, exciting voices or sounds; smoking soon before going to bed; drinking alcohol before going to bed; eating too soon before bedtime; and perhaps falling asleep and napping for awhile before going to bed, removing some of the hormonal influences of deep sleep. Other bad sleep hygiene includes not providing the bedroom conditions conducive to sleep, which include a calm, quiet, relaxing environment with low light; napping too much during the day; and drinking too much coffee or other caffeine containing drinks during the day.

Good sleep hygiene, as indicated in Chapter 5 and Chapter 9, includes maintaining a bedroom environment that is quiet, dark enough, cool enough, and comfortable; going to bed the same time each night or following a ritual that allows enough time for sleep before you need to get up, or that works for you; restricting bedtime activities to sleep or making love; avoiding stimulating activities and exercise right before bedtime; avoiding caffeine drinks after lunch; and avoiding too much alcohol before bedtime. Caffeine has a long biological half-life, so consuming too much caffeine even in the afternoon can adversely affect sleep at night. Too much alcohol consumption before bedtime causes a reduced amount of REM sleep and total sleep, and can cause multiple awakenings after perhaps a short two or three hours of sleep. How much is too much of any of these things depends on an individual's tolerances. Many people find reading in bed makes them fall asleep better, although this is not a recommended activity in bed before turning off the lights. In particular, action-packed books or TV movies should be avoided in the bedroom. Each individual can and should try different ways to find the most effective sleep hygiene for himself, and to adapt them to any changes in schedules or circumstances.

Traveling between time zones also produces sleep problems for many persons, and the frequency of such travel can often be controlled by the individual. As with Phyllis' description of her problem from going and returning over six time zones, her sleep problems were severe for several weeks after the trip. However, this does not suggest the avoidance of interesting or necessary travel as needed or desired; the benefits of such travel are balanced against the risks of insomnia.

Evening arguments over money, sex, living conditions, or other aspects of personal relationships can also obviously prevent a good night's sleep. These arguments are also under individual control to some extent. Counseling on ways to debate or negotiate, or courses in proper assertiveness can help. Self help can also be obtained from the many books and articles regularly published on such subjects.

In my own case, it took me until late in life to learn that the initial tone of voice can make a big difference. If I am irritated about something and just blurt it out, Phyllis thinks that I am yelling at her. So, before I say something when in this irritated state, I try to take my time and begin my statements with such endearments as, "Dear sweet honey, I would like to say...," or, "My beautiful and dear wife, did you know that when you raise your voice, I often think you are angry at me for something I have done. Could this be so?" Beginning with such endearments often puts my voice into the proper tone. If not, I sometimes just start singing a love song or happy song before talking. One cannot be unhappy when singing a happy song, no matter the ability to carry a tune. Try it. Try to sing a happy tune and see if you can remain angry or unhappy. So, there can be some control over emotions that get you into trouble and cause sleepless nights.

(2) Internal Causes

The causes in number 8 of our questionnaire (presented in the appendix), which has spaces for checkmarks, are comprised mainly of causes over which the individual has little or no control. Without some kind of treatment or remedy, sleep apnea is a symptom that the individual might not be aware of when sleeping; he is told about it after he is awake. Respiratory problems, transient or chronic, can be due to infections or impairments beyond the individual's control. Pain might not be suppressed by over-the-counter medications and, if it is due to some physical defect or disease, can be alleviated only by medical treatment. Depression, anxiety, and excessive worry over sleep loss might be helped only by appropriate medical or psychotherapeutic treatments. The parasomnias (disorders that are associated with sleep and can adversely affect sleep), such as screaming in sleep (night terrors), sleepwalking, and violent acts, are not under the individual's control; if repetitious and serious, they also require medical help. Menopausal symptoms, or effects of pregnancy, may often be helped by comfort measures, such as the use of soft pillows and warm baths.

All of these internal causes have appeared in one or another of the persons who responded to our questionnaires, as presented in the narratives of Chapter 6.

(3) Intrinsic Causes Initiated by (1) and (2)

These are the fundamental intrinsic reactions in the brain and glandular systems that cause effects on sleep by physiologic adjustment of the internal hormone secretions that attempt to balance the sleep-wake cycle. The same intrinsic physiologic causes of sound or unsound sleep are initiated by all of the above external causes or internal disorders presented in (1) and (2) above. Initiation of hormone secretions can occur by external stimuli such as bright or dark light, noisy sounds or soft music (or "white noise"), by pain, night terrors, interrupted sleepwalking, or by any other external or internal actions that affect the sleep-wake cycle.

There are two centers at the base of the brain that secrete neurohormones affecting the sleep-wake cycle. One center causes wakefulness and the other induces sleep. The wakefulness center usually dominates, because most of the time we need to be alert for our work or activities, or to protect ourselves from accidents or other hazards. It has also evolved through evolution to protect ourselves and families from danger, or to answer the cry of a baby in distress.

The cells and the hormones they secrete that influence the sleep-wake cycle are referred to as our "biological clocks." Experiments have shown that these clocks would work on a cycle of sleep and wakefulness that would drift to more than 24 hours in the absence of the light and dark times of the day. The influence of daytime and nighttime in an ordinary day results in the biological clock being set to a "circadian rhythm" of 24 hours. This circadian rhythm results in a needed amount of sleep of slightly more than eight hours for the average person, but for some people only six or seven hours may suffice.

The "master clock" is a pea-sized piece of brain tissue consisting of 20,000 cells known as the suprachiasmatic nuclei (SCN). The SCN is located in the hypothalamus, which lies at the base of the brain, just above the crossing of the optic nerves. The SCN is the "awake center." Sunlight stimulates nerve transmission from the retina in the back of our eyes to the SCN. A message is then sent from the SCN to the pituitary gland, which is located in the base of the brain and attached by a stalk to the hypothalamus. The pituitary gland then secretes adrenocorticotrophic hormone (ACTH), which travels to the adrenal glands above the kidney, which then secretes cortisol. Cortisol and other hormones are responsible for body metabolism. In addition, one of the functions of cortisol is to keep our body alert during the day.

Thus, when cortisol is secreted, if we have had sufficient sleep the night before, we become alert during the day. Greater amounts of cortisol, as well as adrenalin, are secreted when we are in danger or stressed by some fear that is warranted or unwarranted. Phyllis has described her fear upon waking in the middle of the night of not getting adequate sleep, the fear in turn producing the cortisol and adrenalin that cause the negative feedback of further wakefulness, and thus the inability to get back to sleep without the help of some sleep medication.

The pineal gland, located near the hypothalamus and pituitary gland, secretes melatonin. Secretion of melatonin is stimulated by darkness, relaxation, and quiet, and is responsible for helping us fall asleep. Melatonin ceases to be produced when sufficient light enters the room. This explains the difficulties of jet lag or working some night shifts, which tinker with the biological clock, which in turn needs to be reset to a normal circadian rhythm. This resetting can take time, and can result in a transient insomnia that can last up to weeks.

It is hoped that this brief recapitulation of the neurological pathways and hormonal secretions that affect the sleep-wake cycle provide an understanding of the secondary intrinsic causes of insomnia that might help the reader who suffers from inadequate sleep. As is well known, understanding of a source of distress can often reduce the stress.

Table of Causes of Sleep Loss

A table of causes of sleep loss found in the questionnaires is now presented below to offer further insights about the most frequent causes of sleep loss. These causes have been divided into only seven categories for feasibility of examining causes of interest to the reader, and to provide a way for the reader to match his own concerns to those of questionnaire respondents. In this way, the reader may find narratives of most interest and most likely helpful to his own sleep problems.

Table of Causes of Sleep Loss Found in Questionnaires

The following table uses the following inserted letters to indicate whether, or how much, each cause on the top line impairs the sleep of each questionnaire responder whose narrative number is in the left hand column: NI—no information or not listed as a cause, SC—a most serious cause, CC—a contributing cause together with others, NC—not a serious cause, as indicated by specific information on the respondent's questionnaire. The inserting of these letters required judgments again about frequency and severity, just as did the placement of narratives into symptom categories in Chapter 6.

Narrative number	Beyond control: partner noise; work schedules	Worry or stress	Pain preventing sleep	Obstructive sleep apnea (OSA) or respiratory problems	Restless leg or periodic limb movement syndromes	Medical disorder	Psychiatric disorder
1	NI	CC	CC	NI	NI	NI	NI
2	NI	CC	NI	NI	NI	NI	NI
3	CC	CC	NI	NI	NI	NI	NI
4	NI	NI	NI	NI	NI	NI	NI
5	NI	CC	NI	NI	NI	NI	NI
6	NI	NI	NC	NI	NI	NI	NI
7	NI	NI	NI	NI	NI	CC	NI
8	CC	CC	NI	CC	NI	NI	NI
9	NI	NI	NI	CC	NI	NI	NI
10	NI	CC	NI	NI	NI	NI	NI
11	NI	CC	NI	NI	NI	NI	NI
12	NI	CC	NI	NI	NI	NI	NI
13	NI	NI	NI	CC	NI	CC	NI
14	SC	CC	NI	NI	NI	NI	NI
15	SC	CC	CC	CC	NI	NI	NI
16	NI	CC	NI	NI	NI	NI	NI
17	NI	CC	CC	NI	CC	NI	NI
18	NI	NI	NI	NC	NI	NI	NI
19	NC	NC	NI	NI	NI	NI	NI
20	NI	CC	CC	CC	CC	CC	NI
21	NI	NI	NI	NI	NI	NI	NI
22	NI	CC	NI	NI	CC	NI	NI
23	SC	CC	NI	NI	CC	NI	NI
24	SC	NC	NI	NI	NI	NI	NI
25	NI	NI	NI	NI	NI	NI	NI
26	SC	NI	NI	NI	NI	NI	NI
27	NC	CC	NI	NI	NI	NI	NI
28	CC	SC	CC	NI	CC	NI	NI
29	NI	NI	NI	NI	NI	NI	NI
30	CC	NI	NI	NI	NI	NI	NI
31	SC	CC	NI	NI	NI	NI	NI
32	CC	NI	NI	NI	NI	NI	NI
33	NI	CC	NI	NI	NI	NI	NI
34	SI	SI	SC	SC	SC	NI	SC
35	NI	NI	NI	CC	NI	NI	NI
36	NI	SC	NI	NI	NI	NI	NI
37	NI	CC	NI	NI	NI	CC	NI
38	NC	NI	NI	NI	NI	NI	NI
39	NI	NI	NI	NI	NI	NI	NI
40	NI	NI	NI	NI	NI	NI	NI
41	NI	NI	NI	NI	NC	NI	NI
42	NI	SC	SC	NI	CC	CC	NI

Observations from Table of Causes

Those in the sample who show an entire row of NI are ones who have listed no sleep complaints at all. They represent the best sleepers, by this observation as well as the information given in their questionnaires. These persons with an entire row of NI represent about 20 percent of the sample.

Those columns with all NI except one that is not a serious SC cause bring the all NI group up to about half the sample, which is consistent with the finding in Chapter 6, counting all of the first category and half of the second, as persons not having serious problems with insomnia. This result is also consistent with the observation that one-third to one-fifth of the adult populations have some symptoms of insomnia in the U.S. and Western nations.[5]

Only one person in our sample has indicated seeking psychiatric diagnoses and treatment. Four have sought medical help, including those given a prescription that provided help with sleep. Thus, a total of five out of this sample have sought and received medical assistance. Although statistical uncertainty in such a small number is large, the number is consistent with the report that 10 to 15 percent of the population have a serious problem with insomnia, requiring general medical or psychiatric assistance.[6]

In addition to suggestions in Chapter 6 for using narratives to consider ways others relieve sleep problems, the reader may also use the table on previous page. By reviewing only narratives that have SC in their rows, the reader who has serious problems with insomnia can locate the brief narratives of interest in Chapter 6 and examine the tried remedies and treatments. Readers with less serious but significant problems may examine narratives having two or more boxes with CC and/or NC that match up to the causes of their insomnias. The most frequent external causes are shown in the cartoon of Exhibit 3 on the next page.

Persons might also wish to examine, from the table of remedies below, the narratives of persons using remedies of interest for relieving the person's particular sleep problems.

Effects of Sleep Loss

The most frequent adverse effects of sleep loss found among our sample of questionnaire respondents in Chapter 6 may be represented by the last four complaints, 7 to 10 of Neubauer. However, as also noted previously in Chapter 6, we have had to modify these complaints so that if they are not

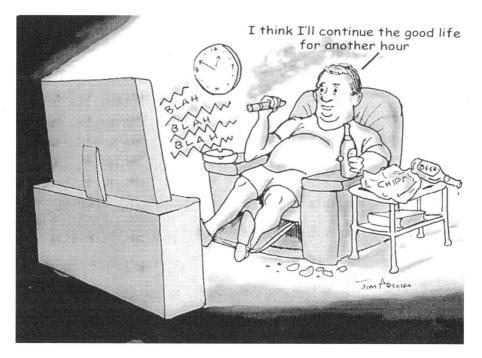

Exhibit 3. Illustration of Poor Sleep Hygiene. A cross should be across this picture to illustrate some BAD causes of poor sleep that must be forbidden to have good sleep hygiene.

experienced all of the time indicated, they might still be serious enough to the individual to cause significant adverse effects at least some of the time. Thus, we may rewrite these complaints as (7) having trouble getting out of bed in the morning in time to get to work or meet an obligation; (8) not feeling rested enough to perform adequately most of the time; (9) usually feeling fatigued most of the day after losing sleep; and (10) almost never being able to take a refreshing nap.

In Chapter 6 for both men and women, we placed those having sleep problems that caused some degree of suffering, but which are managed to prevent serious consequences most of the time, into the category of "living with" insomnia; those having sleep problems and having "concerns or difficulties" that appeared to cause serious consequences most of the time were placed in the third category. In this way, we counted half of the persons in the second categories of men and women, and all in the third, as having insomnia for comparison with the statistics in the earlier chapters.

In this way, we extended the Neubauer definition of insomnia: (1) having sleep problems and (2) suffering from them. The number 2 in this definition was thus divided into those who suffered significantly but seemed to live adequately with insomnia, and those who suffered so seriously that major adverse effects on life occurred. The judgments of whether a responder should be placed in the "living with" category or the third more serious category of insomnia were made from the information on the questionnaire, as presented in the narratives of Chapter 6. Estimating the frequency of insomnia in the above way, half from the second category of our narratives and all from more serious category resulted in the agreements with published statistics on the proportions of the population suffering from insomnia, as concluded in the latter paragraphs of Chapter 6.

All of the complaints 7 to 10 of Neubauer have been found in the persons responding to our questionnaires, as observed in Chapter 6. Also, Chapter 3 will show that Phyllis and I have experienced all of these effects to some degree, except that I am able to take naps for a couple of hours, or short rests of fifteen or twenty minutes in an alpha state, so that I can regain enough energy to continue what I need to do during my planned work or activity hours.

We believe that the vast majority of our readers will find that their sleep problems are represented by the categories of Neubauer, and that they can find among the numbered list of narratives in Chapter 6 those that match up with sleep complaints of their own. In this way, readers may read narratives that present effects of insomnia similar to their own and perhaps find ways that others have "lived with," or dealt with, their problems.

In addition to feelings of tiredness or exhaustion, sleep deprivation can result in mood changes or depression that can affect physical or mental health. Long-term insomnia can have adverse effects on a person's quality of life, health, and economics. Chronic insomniacs have experienced irritability, clinical depression, decreased ability to concentrate, memory lapses, decreased productivity, and more missed work days. Not only do chronic insomniacs risk poor health, they also risk death or injury from accidents at work, on the road, in the air, and on the sea.

Restorative processes in deep sleep, described in Chapter 8, include regulation of the immune systems of the body. The immune system provides certain white cells, macrophages that clean up debris, and antibodies, which fight infections and other ailments. As noted in Chapter 8, college students who choose an excess of social as well as study activities at the cost of adequate sleep have a much higher incidence of colds, mononucleosis, and other infections. Medical interns and residents, also known to be overworked and sleep deprived, have a higher incidence of colds, flu, and other diseases. A healthy immune system is also known to reduce the incidence of cancer. These diseases are among the more serious effects of sleep loss. Medical and nursing personnel who are sleep deprived have also been responsible for mistakes in hospitals that have caused injury or death. The medical and hospital organizations are attempting to correct this situation.

The shorter duration of sleep within Western societies has also been correlated with increase incidence of type 2 diabetes. Insulin sensitivity is not fixed even in healthy persons, so even one night of lost sleep causes insulin resistance, a component of type 2 diabetes. Sleep deprivation can also lead to heart disease, strokes, high blood pressure, kidney disease, and metabolic diseases. Insufficient sleep can also reduce growth in the young, and impede tissue repair after injury. Chapter 8 has provided examples and stories about how these detrimental effects of sleep have resulted in injury, death, and billions of dollars of economic loss in even our most advanced societies.

Remedies for Improving Sleep and Their Associated Effectiveness

Chapter 9 reviews in some detail the remedies for improving sleep. The remedies can be divided into three categories for this summary: self-help remedies; prescribed or over-the-counter (OTC) medications; and treatments requiring sleep center examinations and specialized medical management. Any of these remedies will vary in effectiveness depending on an individual's constitution and life situation.

Self-Help Remedies

The first self-help remedies that should be tried are the reversal of the bad sleep hygiene practices listed at the beginning of this chapter; convert your habits to good sleep hygiene. Generally, avoid more than a couple of ounces of alcohol in the evening within a couple of hours of going to bed, or even avoid alcohol altogether if you are more sensitive to its waking effects after going to sleep. Do not eat much within the last few hours of going to bed, and cut down on the fat calories. (I [Allen] once adopted the habit of not eating or drinking after about 7 P.M., and had my best sleep experiences during those good habit changes.) Do not drink more than a couple of cups of coffee during the day, and try to stay away from coffee or other caffeine-containing drinks after noon. As indicated in Chapter 9, caffeine has a long half-life in the systemic circulation. Try to get to bed so that you can have eight hours of sleep or at least three to four hours of sleep and peaceful rest and thought before arising. See the most frequent bad sleep hygiene practices in the cartoon of the preceding subsection.

Sondra Kornblatt's recent book, *Restful Insomnia*, cited in the notes sections, provides many self-help remedies with recommendations of steps for applying them.[7] The physician, Teresa E. Jacobs, M.D., who wrote Kornblatt's Foreword and who herself manages a sleep center, writes, "Her book can help those with frequent insomnia explore different techniques at their own pace and focus on the ones that seem most beneficial." We agree with Dr. Jacobs. After describing common remedies in use, Kornblatt describes a vast number of naturopathic and other remedies that can be tried, in addition to those provided in other references or centers. She focuses on combining mind, body, and spirit to avoid worry about sleep and practice ways of utilizing the time in bed to obtain adequate rest and renewed energy. Some of the remedies in the book have been used to find relief from sleeplessness by Phyllis and me. We have found that massage of the head and shoulders can relieve headaches that prevent sleep. I used this morning, while Phyllis slept, to massage my scalp and face with certain amounts of pressure and motion as learned about 30 years ago in an evening massage class, to relieve tensions that prevented my going to sleep. Sometimes I massage Phyllis' head and shoulders to relieve pains resulting from her vigorous exercise program, so she can relax and more easily fall asleep. Many other remedies are described in Kornblatt's book, if none of those in Chapter 9 are effective.

Prescribed or Over-the-Counter (OTC) Medications

The use of prescribed or OTC medications (sleeping pills) are often effective but sometimes can become addictive to certain people, as described in Chapter 9 and other sections of this book. Many persons will not allow themselves to experiment with such medications because they are concerned about such addictions. Many of these medications also have undesirable side effects, particularly when attention is not paid to warnings in the packaged inserts, or when self-medications are not monitored by a personal physician. Phyllis has described in Chapter 3 how an initial medication she was taking caused great stress and nearly resulted in harmful effects, until a psychiatrist changed her prescriptions, followed up by further management by our family doctor. Try to make sure, if you do experiment with any OTC sleeping pills, that at some point you obtain professional monitoring. Often, the pharmacists at drug stores can provide important advice and assistance.

Some overview of medications taken by others can be obtained by reading the narratives in Chapter 6 of persons who have sleep complaints similar to your own. Narratives with complaints similar to yours can be found in the numbered list of narratives following the italicized individual narratives and the complaint list of Neubauer in Chapter 6.

Treatments Requiring Sleep Center Examinations and/or Medical Management

Dr. David Neubauer, in his book *Understanding Sleeplessness*, cited in the chapter notes, has clearly and relatively concisely explained the nature of sleep center tests and diagnostics, in addition to defining the various complaints and treatments for insomnia.[8] Other books cited in the notes also can help in obtaining an understanding of when this more intensive kind of medical diagnosis is needed. If neither the self-help nor medication remedies alleviate serious sleep problems, the sufferer should consider the need for a referral to a sleep center managed by physicians certified in the appropriate specialties. Treatment in these centers will usually result in final remedies for insomnia.

Variations in Effectiveness

As indicated in the beginning paragraph of this third section of the chapter, the effectiveness of any remedy for insomnia can vary from time to time, or over various stages of life. Phyllis has described in Chapter 3 how she usually takes only one capsule each night of doxepin (a small dose) before she goes to sleep at 9 or 9:30 P.M. Sometimes, however, if the doxepin seems ineffective and she wakes up without being able to fall back to sleep, she then might fall back on Ambien. Allen had no problems with allergies that kept him awake until his late 30s; he thought he was Superman in that regard. Then allergies hit him, and for years he needed to take an OTC medication. It is difficult to fall asleep when one's nose is running or sneezing. When he first sought the proper medication, he found that all the remedies used by his friends did not work for him. After trying various medications in the drug stores, he finally found that Actifed delivered relief.

So, if you find a remedy but then it ceases to work after awhile, try other remedies or further consultation with your doctor. Remedies for insomnia might well vary in effectiveness through your life stages. You might need to do one-animal research and try many other remedies as some become ineffective. However, that one animal is you, the most important animal in your own research. You alone might turn out to be your best healthcare provider.

However, you should always check your changes in remedies with your doctor. Many remedies have side effects that also vary with the individual and over life stages.

Further Analysis of Narratives in Chapter 6 from Sleep Questionnaires

In addition to the observations in Chapter 6, a further tabular analysis of remedy categories, similar to that used with the Table of Causes above, is also based on data in the sleep questionnaires data. This remedy tabulation is provided and examined to both give the reader another way to examine particular scenarios that compare to his own and might provide insights for improving sleep; and provide another overview of sleep problems and solutions that might pertain to friends and family members.

For his own benefit, it should not take much time for any reader to match up a responder's characteristics with his own. For characteristics of interest according to the letters in the table, the reader needs just to find the numbered narrative to find the age, sex, and other characteristics in the narrative. The examination of a numbered narrative in Chapter 6 should take only a matter of seconds to determine whether it is in the reader's interest.

Table of Remedies Found in Questionnaires

The table below uses the following inserted letters to represent how remedies have been tried to remove positive or negative influences on sleep: E—tried and effective, E&NN—effective when needed but not always needed, TN—tried, not effective, A—against trying, B—bad sleep hygiene, NC— no control (e.g., prevented by partner or circumstances), NI—no information given on questionnaire, NN—not needed, NT—not tried

Narrative number	Good sleep hygiene	No coffee, food or > 2 oz. of alcohol in evening	No stimulating TV or scary books in bed	Make up for sleep loss with naps	OTC or prescriptions used for sleep	Medical help and/or sleep center tests
1	NI	NI	NI	NI	A	NN
2	NI	NI	NI	NI	E	NI
3	NC	NI	E	E	A	NN
4	E	NI	E	NN	NN	NN
5	NI	NI	NI	NI	NT	NN
6	E	NI	E	NN	E&NN	NN

Narrative number	Good sleep hygiene	No coffee, food or > 2 oz. of alcohol in evening	No stimulating TV or scary books in bed	Make up for sleep loss with naps	OTC or prescriptions used for sleep	Medical help and/or sleep center tests
7	NI	NI	NI	NI	E	E
8	E	NI	NI	NI	E	NN
9	NT	NI	NI	E	NT	NN
10	E	NI	NI	NI	E	NN
11	NT	NT	NI	NI	E	E
12	NT	NT	E	NI	NT	NN
13	NI	NI	NT	E	E	NT
14	NT	NI	NI	NI	E	NT
15	NT	NI	NI	NI	TN	E
16	TN	NI	NI	NI	E	NN
17	TN	NI	NI	NI	E	E
18	NI	NI	NI	E	NN	NN
19	NT	NI	NI	E	E	NN
20	NI	NI	NI	NI	NT	TN
21	NI	NI	NI	E	NN	NN
22	NT	NI	NI	NI	TN	NN
23	NC	NI	NI	NI	NT	NT
24	E	NI	E	NI	NN	NN
25	NI	NI	NI	E	NN	NN
26	NC	NI	NI	NC	NN	NN
27	NT	NI	NI	NI	E	NN
28	NI	NI	NI	TN	A, E	NN
29	NI	NI	NI	MM	NN	NN
30	E	NI	E	NI	NT	NT
31	NC	NI	E	NI	TN	NN
32	E	NI	E	NI	NT	NT
33	NT	NI	B	NI	E	NN
34	NI	NI	E	NI	E	E
35	NN	NI	E	NI	NT	E
36	NI	NI	NI	NI	NN	NN
37	NT	NI	NI	NI	NT	NT
38	E	NI	E	NN	NN	NN
39	NT	NI	NI	NN	E	NN
40	E	E	NI	NN	NN	NN
41	E	E	E	NN	E	NN
42	NI	NI	NI	NI	NT	NI

Some General Observations from the Composite Information in the Table of Remedies

The table shows that in our sample of respondents, those who have serious sleep problems are helped more by prescribed medications or by over-the-counter medications or sleeping pills. Less than half of those helped by sleeping pills were helped by additional medical evaluation and treatment, but some of those who used medication had their prescriptions managed by medical personnel.

Counting the number of Es in the column indicating effectiveness of naps, and looking back to the numbered narratives in Chapter 6, we find that only one of the respondents helped by naps is female, the others are male. This could be considered a statistically significant finding for adult respondents, even from this limited sample, for any nonparametric test. This tells me that Phyllis is not as strange as I thought in not being able to nap during the day. Is the inability of females to nap controlled by a gene in the X chromosome? Some answers to this question might be culled from the exposition of facts in Chapters 2 and 5 that females have more problems than males after puberty and through further ages. In those chapters, the presented effects of hormonal changes and balances also might lend some understanding to this observation of less ability of females to nap during the day.

None of those who were helped in relieving sleep debt by naps appeared to require more intensive medical evaluation and care. Most of them were judged to be in the category of having no serious sleep problems, with some in the category of mild problems and living with insomnia, in the narratives in Chapter 6.

However, we must warn here of the negative effects of naps in affecting the homeostatic balancing of circadium rhythms, making it more difficult after long naps to obtain good sleep during the night. Naps that are short, perhaps 20 minutes or less, can provide additional energy during the day for required activities, without significantly affecting circadian rhythms. Long naps during the day might only contribute to a further listless feeling upon waking, and the loss of daytime hours for productive or recreational activities. Also, long naps use up homeostatic sleep pressure needed to fall asleep at normal bedtime. The effects of napping on sleep experiences are described in much more detail throughout Neubauer's book.

In Phyllis' experience, as indicated in Chapter 3, napping in her adult years has not been a possible remedy for sleep problems. She was last able to take naps sometimes as a teenage counselor in summer camps, when the children under her supervision took naps. Allen's experience confirms the fact that a short nap of less than 20 minutes, or resting for up to that long in the alpha state and with eyes closed, can provide renewed energy for several more hours of productive work or play. He has also experienced lethargy after long naps, and the difficulties of going to sleep at night after such naps.

In regard to sleep hygiene, a review of the narratives in Chapter 6 led to the result in the remedy table that only about 10 cases used good sleep hygiene (the second column in the table), and that about 12 specifically avoided stimulation of TV or reading in bed, in order to improve sleep. However, the significance of these number frequencies is subject to more than random statistical uncertainty; additional uncertainty is due to the judgments of degree of remedy benefit that needed to be made in order to enter Es, or not to enter Es, in most of the cases. It is interesting that only two of the respondents volunteered some information about avoiding excessive eating or drinking within a few hours before bedtime. Other than offering blanks to check for specific causes or parasomnias that at times could adversely affect sleep, as in part 8 of the questions (see appendix), the questionnaire asked only for any other causes that the respondent could attribute to sleep loss.

Allen's experience is that there was a period in earlier life when he adopted the habit of not eating or drinking after about 7 P.M., with bedtimes about 10 P.M., and he had no trouble sleeping soundly, without dreams he could remember, for about six hours on the average. Most of this must have been non–REM sleep. This was in his earlier life when he had to perform well on the job. Now, he is more lackadaisical (or lazy?), lacking willpower (or want power) in his retirement. He often has desserts as well as milk before going to bed. He also tries to get sweet, fattening desserts when out to dinner. Phyllis always watches him and makes him avoid significant ingestion of sugar and fat as much as she can when she is around.

Nevertheless, Allen has also found, in recent years, that he could cease taking Alka-Seltzers or other prescribed medications to relieve heartburn (gastric recycle) after going to bed on a full stomach. A happy discovery in recent years is that he is relieved of heartburn and burps if he gets out of bed, goes to the kitchen after Phyllis is asleep, and instead of taking medications makes an ice-cream soda. He adds several big scoops of highest fat ice cream to half a glass of bubbly soda, lets it fizz, and then slowly downs the good stuff while watching TV. Also, it sure tastes better than the previous remedies. Within the hour, he can then go to bed and sleep without being disturbed by regurgitating food and bubbly burps. This is another of Allen's secrets revealed in this book. Of course, an old man like Allen (and maybe anyone else) must be sure to exercise off the next day or two enough of the calories consumed at night to avoid gaining weight again and having a return of apnea. Nurse Phyllis monitors his blood pressure.

I (Allen) am not just giving out these secrets just to be funny. I once took a course in about 1962 in mathematical modeling of disease prevalence and incidence from a professor Dankward Kodlin. He was a German physician who had taken an interest in mathematical modeling and had come to teach at the Graduate School of Public Health, University of Pittsburgh. In his office one day, Dr. Kodlin told me that he believed that many of the older people who had heart attacks listed on their death certificates were actually victims of eating late at night, lying down, and then returning their food into their lungs and suffocating in their sleep. From my own experiences, and also the loss of some colleagues and friends whose habits I knew, I have been able to accept Dr. Kodlin's theory.

For many years, if I still feel that my food has not been processed and delivered mostly down from my stomach and into the small intestine, and I feel heartburn or reflux to some degree, I take some of my ice-cream soda prescription, and then also beat firmly on my abdomen to shake any food down past any blockage. The beating on my abdomen below the rib cage also helps burp up the carbon dioxide from food digestion, thus allowing further food to digest and pass down into the small intestine. Then, when I feel ready to return to bed, I first will place an extra pillow on the bed to raise my head a bit more. I still remember Dr. Kodlin's scary theory. So far, I am still alive. Ask Phyllis.

A DISCLAIMER: None of the above personal practices of mine are based on careful population research, nor even any significant memory of facts learned in my studies of human biology. I (Allen) just derive them from common sense (my own). Therefore, I accept no responsibility for adverse effects from following any of my recommendations without prior consultation with your physician.

Some words about statistical uncertainties in regard to data in small samples: Readers interested in statistics might appreciate some brief paragraphs about the significance of relative proportions of causes in the data. Now, only those who are interested in and do not despise mathematics should read the paragraphs in this section on statistics.

Suppose we were interested in obtaining something close to a representative sample of the total U.S. population in regard to the sleep experiences and remedies chosen for examination. A survey of the entire national population would be completely outside any financial or organizational possibilities. Thus, within resources that might be provided, a sample of some thousands of persons might be sampled with a carefully prepared and solicited sampling design, to obtain a representative sample of the U.S. population within a demographic range of interest that could offer a dependable response. Then, a sample would be constructed from a population of data in, for example, the National Center of Health Statistics, in such a way that each individual in the U.S. in the selected demographic range for the study would have an equal probability (chance) of being included in our "representative" sample.

With a limited size population sample, the chances (probabilities) of persons appearing in a particular pattern among a category of causes would occur according to what is called a "multinomial distribution," a mathematical formula made up of products of the underlying probabilities of the causes of insomnia that actually are present in the U.S. population. The distribution of occurrences of a particular symptom, effect, or other characteristic would occur according to a "binomial distribution." Of course, the exact underlying frequencies in the entire population (i.e., the United States adults over 21 years of age) are not usually known in population studies (even the census has uncertainties); otherwise we would not need to have collected our sample of data.

These frequencies, in our study or any other, can only be estimated, in turn, from the number counted for each cause in our sample data. With a large enough population and only the limited number of letter descriptions used, each letter could be expected to occur below a cause according to an approximate Poisson distribution, to which a binomial distribution converges for large enough study population. For about 25 counts of a particular letter, the probability envelope of the discrete Poisson distribution would very roughly begin to approach what is commonly called, in elementary statistics courses, a continuous "normal distribution" or, as known by physicists, "Gaussian distribution." Let us assume for simplicity in illustrating statistical uncertainty that the normal distribution of occurrence of a cause (say, the number of those with non–NIs below the worry-stress heading in the table of causes [i.e., the number of those who do not indicate that worry has anything to do with their insomnia]) has been adequately approached for our purposes. Then, for example, the true underlying frequency of non–NIs in the total U.S. population would be 68 percent likely to be in a range of plus or minus one standard deviation about the frequency observed in our sample. The standard deviation for about 25 non–NIs could be approximated roughly, for a count of 25 or more in the category, to the square root of the number, as the probability envelope approaches the normal from the Poisson.

Thus, if 25 non–NIs (those whose sleep is at least somewhat affected by worry or stress) are counted in the "worry or stress" column, we might have about 68 percent confidence that the true U.S. frequency of non–NIs would for our sample be estimated to be in the range 25±5 (since 5 is the square root of 25, i.e., $5 \times 5 = 25$). Thus, we could bet 68 dollars to 32 dollars that the true average number of persons, whose sleep is affected by worry-stress in a large number of surveys the same size of ours, would be between 20 and 30 persons. This would be a fair bet and both betters would come out about even after betting on many such surveys.

If the person betting 68 dollars on the range of the average number of non–Ns was told that the 68 percent confidence interval was, say 22 to 27, he would likely lose money after betting on many surveys.

These paragraphs are presented only to give the reader a simplified view of how the range of statistical uncertainty is calculated. A more exact analysis would be much too lengthy for the purposes of this book. If less than about 25, the 68 percent interval as described above would deviate much more than obtained using the square root of the number observed. For a much greater number of non–NIs in a survey of persons even far greater than the number of non–Ns observed, the confidence interval calculations could be more closely approximated by a normal distribution, and then a 95-percent interval could be estimated from the number of non–Ns plus or minus two standard deviations.

Many readers might not want to spend much time thinking about the above paragraphs on statistics, so if they are not worthwhile, cross them out in your book (if you own it). An additional picture of statistical uncertainty referring to the Table of Remedies: Readers interested in statistics might again appreciate some discussion about the significance of relative proportions in data categories in the Table of Remedies, following that above for the Table of Causes above.

Here we will just provide another story to help visualize the meaning of "confidence intervals" in statistics.

Suppose two billionaires each took a million dollars to Las Vegas to be available for gambling, and were betting on the number of times a slot machine with the six notations at the top of the slide would turn up an E in the fifth column. Assume, as after the Table of Causes, that 25 is the true underlying average number of Es to come up under a column, and the standard deviation is the square root of 25, which is 5.

In a first casino where they gamble, the number of times particular letters would come up would be governed by wheels designed to contain letters as they would be in the entire U.S. population (assuming the frequencies were known exactly to the designers, but not to the players). One bet would be made on 100 rolls (taking a few minutes). One of the billionaire players would bet 68 dollars that Es would come up in a particular column between 20 and 30 times out of the 100 rolls; the other better would bet 32 dollars that the number would not be between 20 and 30. If this game of 100 rolls were played for 8 hours each day for, say, five days (hundreds of plays), then we would have a fair bet situation. Each player would end up winning about half the time, and losing half the time. At the end of five days, each player would have about the same amount of money left of the original million dollars he allotted for the week's gambling.

However, if they had entered a second casino, where the designer of the slot machine had placed fewer Es on that column of the wheel, so that there would be less than 68 percent chance, say only 65 percent chance of an E coming up between 20 and 30 times in the column for 100 rolls, then the player betting on between 20 and 30 appearing would eventually lose more than the one betting outside 20 and 30. This is the way in Las Vegas that gambling machines can be designed to ensure eventual profits to the casino owner, while giving the impression of at least a reasonable chance to win in a limited series of tries.

Perhaps this short statistical tirade of the author will be of interest to the reader. If not, as indicated after the statistical paragraphs following the Table of Causes, scratch out these paragraphs with a black permanent marker pen. I hope that, for some readers who might never have studied statistical methods, it might help understand somewhat the uncertainties in our discussions of the proportions of data in certain categories.

CHAPTER 11

Conclusions and Recommendations

At this point we hope you have learned much about insomnia, other sleep disorders, causes and remedies. Perhaps you can relate to our personal stories and those who have so graciously shared their stories with us. Most of us are aware that if we obtain insufficient sleep, we don't feel our best during daytime hours (or nighttime if we do shift work). We know we can be most productive if we do get sufficient sleep, according to our special needs. For those of you who do have insomnia or other sleep disorder, you probably have felt the troublesome effects of sleep deprivation.

How much sleep we require in order to feel good and be most productive in our lives does vary from person to person, depending on one's particular biological clock and lifestyle. However, the phenomenon of sleep remains much of a mystery, as it has been in times past. REM sleep is particularly fascinating. Dreams have probably puzzled mankind for centuries. Freud had his psychoanalytic theories about the meaning of dreams, which have been disregarded by modern theorists. They still remain a mystery to many of us. REM sleep disorders and other parasomnias can be disturbing to the sufferer or his or her family members. There are remedies that will conquer these problems in many instances.

It is still puzzling that so many people—as revealed by surveys and our own data—suffer from insomnia or other sleep disorders. When we have talked with acquaintances about our book, many have revealed they have insomnia or other sleep disturbance. During these discussions, we have asked people if they would consider completing our questionnaire. This was one way we gathered our data, as explained earlier. As summarized in Chapter 10, it is interesting that many of their stories are consistent with many of the

166

situations and underlying problems described in the books and articles we have cited. We hope that the composites of information in Chapter 10 will provide a concise review of causes and possible remedies for insomnia.

It seems that the invention of the electric light bulb was the culprit, in many cases, that started the problem of sleep disturbances. Prior to this remarkable invention, people just ceased working and retired to bed as darkness approached and then got up at the crack of dawn to begin their chores and start a new day. Of course, we really don't know what sleep problems people might have experienced before the advent of artificial light, since this issue wasn't addressed historically. Perhaps some people did have "innate" insomnias with possible genetic predisposition or other sleep disorders described in Chapters 5 and 7. But sleep problems were not recognized as health issues until the 1950s, when, according to Dr. William Dement, sleep study and sleep medicine arrived on the scene.

The reader should consider improvements in light conditions and other sleep hygiene if these might alleviate personal habits that are interfering with sleep.

As shown throughout this book, many people suffer from sleeplessness, disturbed sleep, or other specific sleep disorders. As revealed in our own stories and those of the people we surveyed, some people cope with their problems and others have sought help. Of those who are troubled, some have learned to live with insomnia and some have sought medical attention.

It is interesting that, of the people we surveyed who had expressed sleep problems, more were troubled by poor sleep maintenance than by sleep onset problems. Many would have little difficulty in going to sleep, but would wake up in the wee hours of the morning (e.g., 2 to 4 A.M.) and not be able to go back to sleep, or would be awake for two or more hours.

The cause or causes of your sleep problems might elude you. For example, if you have an underlying sleep disorder, such as sleep apnea, you might not be aware of the problem. (Check Phyllis's experience with Allen in Chapter 3.) However, if your bed partner has trouble sleeping because of your loud snoring or gasping, he or she will likely tell you so. Believe him or her and seek medical treatment, or treat yourself in some way like losing weight— as Allen did. He no longer snores.

Obstructive sleep apnea is one common problem that might require diagnosis and treatment in a sleep laboratory, if self-help does not work. Other disorders that might be best diagnosed and treated in a sleep lab by sleep specialists are also described in Chapters 5 and 7. There are known effective remedies for most of these problems.

Remember that sleep patterns change with age. Arthritic pains and other pains, emotional and psychiatric problems, and other disorders that increase with age might not be susceptible to self-help, and might require medical identification and treatment.

There are several treatment options, including those available for self-help that are covered in Chapter 9. Basically there are three modes of treatment: (1) medications, be it by prescription, over-the-counter remedies, or herbal preparations; (2) psychotherapies; and (3) alternative methods. One alternative method is meditation—learning how to rest your mind.

Both of us (Allen and Phyllis) know how our active minds prevent us, at times, from obtaining needed sleep. Our minds are often active trying to solve problems, worrying about family or world issues, or thinking about projects we are working on. I (Phyllis) worry about many things, including sleep (as described in our stories in Chapter 3). The challenge for us and for others in similar circumstances is to learn how to quiet our minds, or relax and use them constructively when we cannot sleep.

John Selby, in his book *Secrets of a Good Night's Sleep*, tells how to do this through meditation. He states, "The main object of this meditation is to gently move your awareness out of chronic thinking patterns and emotional contractions, and into a deeper awareness of your body here in the present moment."[1] Selby takes you step by step through the process of meditation. Selby's and Kornblatt's (*Restful Insomnia*) books are excellent resources that not only help you live with insomnia, but provide ways to quiet your mind to help you obtain a more restful night's sleep.

Our main conclusions and recommendations for relief from sleep problems according to age group are:

• In regard to infants whose sleep patterns are a problem to their parents, not only to them, we recommend examining the more recent books on sleep solutions for infants. We especially favor the book, listed in the notes, by Elizabeth Pantley, *The No-Cry Sleep Solution: Gentle Ways to Help Your Baby Sleep Through the Night*, because it is consistent with our personal experiences with six infants. Summary suggestions for relieving infant sleep problems are provided in the pages of our *Living with Insomnia* book, and may be tried at first. However, Pantley's book provides the many useful procedures and forms for carrying out recommended procedures for gently leading an infant as early as possible into sleep patterns pleasant to the entire family. Her own physician has written a foreword in this book that indicates he gives this book to parents to help with managing their children's sleep problems as well as their own. The reader might also wish to consult the book by the Durand in order to examine a physician's discussion and recommendations for remedies and treatments for children's sleep problems. Durand's book is also a fairly recent book that will provide additional references for those who would like to study this issue further.

Our personal experiences support the above references. As described in Chapter 4, Allen managed to put each of his three children to sleep without letting them cry interminably. He believed that newborns have no desire just to irritate their parents. Rather than letting a baby just cry to sleep, Allen would pick up his baby, cuddle him, dance with him, and give him enough firm pats on the back to burb up the gas bubbles that were causing pain or preventing needed sleep. Then, Allen would lay the baby down, massage its back gently, and sing a peaceful song such as, "I'll Be Loving You Always," repeatedly and more softly each time until the baby fell asleep. With each repetition of the song, softer massages turning into light caresses were employed. In this way, Allen was able to bring each of his infants into good sleep habits within a few weeks or months. As also described in Chapter 4, Phyllis has had successful experiences leading her children into pleasant sleeping patterns within the first few months after birth, without usually needing to let them "cry it out." Thus, both Phyllis' and Allen's experiences are consistent with those of Pantley, and we highly recommend obtaining a copy of her book for use throughout the early stages of your child's life.

- For children as they pass into their early years and later, Durand's book and the included references provides a fairly recent review of successful ways of helping a child build good sleep habits. We have some suggestions in earlier chapters, but if they do not work, a book like Durand's should be consulted. We personally recommend limiting a child's usage of violent video games or watching violent TV shows until late into the night, as some parents do. Children need some discipline in order to develop good sleep habits that will allow better performance in school or at play.

- For students in the teenage years, the parents can only coax the children to adopt good sleep hygiene and habits. Often, some of them might need extra time for evening study if they are pursuing especially advanced high school curricula. If in college, the parents usually have little control over late night study and/or partying. As indicated in Chapter 3 and elsewhere, all we could do with our grandchildren is give them gentle, loving advice. Fortunately, despite their often poor sleep in college, two of them are still alive and healthy after recent graduation, and are moving ahead into their careers.

- For adults past the age of about 21, in their early years of work or professional activity, their own desire to move ahead in life and achieve success and fulfillment will limit poor sleep habits, because they will soon find with poor sleep habits that they will not be able to advance. For adults, the sleep remedies in Chapter 9, composited in Chapter 10 with the experiences in the narratives as well as integrated with remedies in other chapters, might provide some self-help ideas. If such self-help methods do not work, the reader will be guided in the previous chapters to obtain help from appropriate healthcare professionals.

• For those entering senior or retired status, the pressures of succeeding in life are often over or more subdued. Sleep habits may be adjusted to the desired lifestyle. For those still needing employment, although better sleep habits are needed, these persons have often worked out their own sleep needs, or may consult Chapters 9 and 10 to determine better methods of improving sleep. Often the simple things like trying better applications of the elements of good sleep hygiene, or changing habits of worrying about sleep as described by us in Chapters 3 and 9, or as detailed in Kornblatt's book, will suffice to relieve the suffering from insomnia.

We should also mention here that Kornblatt gives considerable emphasis on spiritual factors that can help improve sleep. Carl Jung, the Swiss psychiatrist who founded many of the original psychoanalytical methods and whose volumes of publication are still available today, found that he often needed to recommend religion and prayer to some of his patients when all other methods failed.[2] Jung was a close associate of Sigmund Freud for six years in the early twentieth century, until they parted over this issue and others. In Chapter 4, Phyllis indicated how insomnia was not considered a medical issue until about 1950. However, the relief from insomnia provided by prayer is mentioned in a few of our questionnaires, and some of the sleep disorders treated by spiritual recommendations of Jung would be similar to many in our samples and in the literature today. I (Allen) can remember that when I was a child, my mother taught me to kneel and pray at the bedside before I went to bed, and that did give me a feeling of peace as I went to sleep. Thus, although we have not dealt with this issue in any detail in this book, we believe that there is much literature and help on this subject from the many clergy available in all communities.

• Otherwise, the reader will learn when appropriate consultation with his healthcare provider is needed. Hopefully this book has provided insight into the causes of your troubled sleep. Understanding the causes of any human ailment is the first step in treating the problem. Oftentimes there are no known underlying causes of insomnia or other sleep disorders. In these situations, it might be helpful to consider the remedies summarized above and discussed in more detail in Chapter 9. Books by other authors, who are authorities on sleep and sleep disorders, are listed in the references for those who might need further help. Some of these books are recent and will themselves include further references for those who wish to study issues of insomnia more deeply. We hope you have found some answers and hope from reading the personal stories and information presented in this book. We wish all of our readers success in alleviating any unique problems and success in conquering or living with insomnia.

Good luck and good night. Allen and I wish you many nights of pleasant sleep.

Appendix:
Questionnaire Package

Questions on Sleep

To: Persons requested to provide information on sleep patterns.
From: Allen and Phyllis Brodsky (Who? See attached brief resumes at end.)

We would like your help in collecting information on sleep problems, including causes, symptoms, effects, treatments, and possible cures. Your input would provide real life stories and information to complement a review of sleep problems in a book, "Living with Insomnia," which we have been contracted to write for McFarland and Company, the publisher of Phyllis' 2008 book, "Control of Childbirth: Women vs. Medicine Through the Ages."

Benefits of Participating:

(1) If you agree to participate in this two-page questionnaire, you will be helping others and possibly yourself to improve sleep habits.

(2) If you provide an e-mail address, we will send you a free draft of our book in 2010. It will include information that might be helpful if you still need improvements in sleep habits.

Confidentiality:

All information will be held confidential; actual names will not be included in the book. You may, or may not, elect to provide a telephone number or other contact information in case we would want to follow up with an interview to obtain additional information, or obtain a select number of stories or scenarios to include in the book. We expect to use a number of stories in the book that might further illustrate important aspects of insomnia.

To complete the survey, you can fill in the form electronically and mail it back to us at *phylbrodsky@msn.com*, or fill it out in paper form and mail it to:

Phyllis L. Brodsky
121 Windjammer Road, Berlin, MD 21811
(For questions: Telephone: 410-641-6523; E-mail:*phylbrodsky@msn.com*)

If you would like to volunteer to be available for questions or an interview, also add your contact information:

Name(s): _____
Address: _____
    Telephone Numbers: Home_____; Cell phone_____
    E-mail: _____

Information and questions for your response (place checkmark where appropriate; provide added information as desired, and use other side or add pages if needed):

Your sex: Male___ Female___
Age as of January 31, 2010 _____
Describe your sleep problems:

Difficulty falling asleep when going to bed. Describe: _____
_____
_____

What time(s) do you usually go to bed? Is bedtime related to sleep problems? Explain: _____
_____

How long do you usually read or engage in other activities before turning off lights? _____

About how long does it take you to fall asleep_____

Waking in the night and not able to go back to sleep: Describe times and hours awake,_____
_____

What time (s) do you want ____or need _____ to get up? _____

Please continue filling out information on the next page.

Do you ever wake up too early and have trouble going back to sleep? Describe approximately your times and hours awake: _____

_____

_____

How do you feel during the day after you have had sleep problems at night? Alert? Tired? Please describe problems. _____

_____

_____

How frequently does your sleep problem occur (in nights per month)?

_____

6. How long have you had sleep problems?
_____weeks, _____months, ____years.

7. Please describe **as far as you can tell**,
Causes of your sleep problems _____

_____

Effects of sleep loss_____

_____

Medical treatments attempted and improvements obtained_____

_____

_____

Self-treatments or over-the-counter pills and improvements_____

_____

_____

Permanent cures? At what ages? _____

_____

_____

Alternative therapies? _____

8. Do have any of the following problems: Sleep apnea___;
Respiratory problems___; Pain___; Restless leg syndrome___;
Depression___; Menopausal symptoms, e.g., night sweats___;
Anxiety___: Talking in your sleep___; Sleep walking___; Nightmares___;
Night terrors___; Violent acts___; Worry over sleep loss____
    Explain or discuss and add any other pertinent information:

_____

_____

_____

Please continue filling out information on the next page.

Narrative (Please provide here, and on additional pages as necessary, a narrative of your experiences with insomnia and related issues. Thanks so much!!)

_____

_____

_____

_____

_____

_____

_____

_____

_____

_____

_____

_____

NOTE AGAIN: ALL INFORMATION WILL REMAIN CONFIDENTIAL. ANY SCENARIOS WILL USE MADE-UP NAMES.

Date Completed by Participant: _____

February 22, 2010

To: Participants in providing interviews and/or completed questionnaires in insomnia

Allen and I are writing a book on LIVING WITH INSOMNIA, under contract to McFarland Publishers. They have requested that we get signed permission to use quotes from interviews or information provided in questionnaires, even though all information submitted to us will be kept totally confidential, will be filed by number, and no names will be connected with information entered into our book or used in any other way.

Please read the statement below and sign, and print your signature and date below the statement below. Attach this or enclose it with the information you have sent or presented.

Sincerely,
Phyllis and Allen Brodsky

Permission is granted for use of the information and/or interview that I have provided, either in the book to be published on insomnia (with final title to be established by McFarland) provided that my name is not used or connected with any information provided in interviews or on questionnaire forms, or delivered to you, the authors, in any other way.

*Signature*_____

*Printed name*_____

*Printed title*_____

*Date*_____

Chapter Notes

Chapter 1

1. David N. Neubauer, *Understanding Sleeplessness: Perspectives on Insomnia* (Baltimore: The Johns Hopkins University Press, 2003), 1–18.

2. Mary Brophy Marcus, "Americans of All Races Don't Get Enough Sleep," *USA Today*, March 8, 2010.

3. Carlos H. Schenck, *Sleep. A Groundbreaking Guide to the Mysteries, the Problems, and the Solutions* (New York: Avery, 2007), 17.

4. Neubauer, *Understanding Sleeplessness*, 1–6.

5. M.J. Sateia, K. Doghramji, P.J. Hauri, and C.M. Morin, "Evaluation of Chronic Insomnia," *An American Academy of Sleep Medicine Review* 23, no. 2 (2000): 1–65.

6. J. Paul Caldwell, *Sleep: A Complete Guide to Sleep Disorders and a Better Night's Sleep* (Buffalo, NY: Firefly Books, 2003), 84–85.

7. Sateia, et al., "Evaluation of Chronic Insomnia."

8. David Neubauer, "Can't Sleep? What to Know About Insomnia," *National Sleep Foundation*, www.sleepfoundation.org/article/sleep-related-problems/insomnia-and-sleep.

9. Meir H. Kryger, *A Woman's Guide to Sleep Disorders* (New York: McGraw-Hill, 2004), xi.

10. Schenck, *Sleep*, 14.

11. C. Ruhl, "Sleep Is a Vital Sign," *Nursing for Women's Health* 14, no. 3 (2010): 243–247.

12. William C. Dement, *The Promise of Sleep* (New York: Dell, 1999), 60.

13. Kryger, *A Woman's Guide to Sleep Disorders*, 3.

14. Dement, *The Promise of Sleep*, 98–99.

15. Stanley Coren, *Sleep Thieves* (New York: Free Press Paperbacks, 1996), 1–2.

16. Schenck, *Sleep*, 13.

Chapter 2

1. William C. Dement, *The Promise of Sleep* (New York: Dell, 1999), 17.

2. D.T. Max, "The Secrets of Sleep," *National Geographic* (May 2010): 76.

3. Ibid., 77.

4. Meir H. Kryger, *A Woman's Guide to Sleep Disorders* (New York: McGraw-Hill, 2004), 7–8.

5. David N. Neubauer, *Understanding Sleeplessness: Perspectives on Insomnia* (Baltimore: The Johns Hopkins University Press, 2003), 39.

6. "Circadian Rhythm—Keeping Time," *National Institute of General Medical Sciences*, May 15, 2010, www.nigms.nih.gov/publications/factsheet_circadian-rhythms.htm.

7. Max, "The Secrets of Sleep."

8. "Circadian Rhythm—Keeping

Time," *National Institute of General Medical Sciences*, May 15, 2010, www.nigms.nih.gov/publications/factsheet_circadian-rhythms.htm.

9. J. Paul Caldwell, *Sleep: A Complete Guide to Sleep Disorders and a Better Night's Sleep* (Buffalo, NY: Firefly Books, 2003), 20–21.

10. Neubauer, *Understanding Sleeplessness*, 24–25.

11. R. Kuller, "The Influence of Light on Circarhythms in Humans," *Journal of Physiological Anthropology and Applied Human Science* 21, no. 2 (2002): 87–91.

12. Ibid.

13. Caldwell, *Sleep*, 30–33.

14. C. Drake, "Shift Work and Sleep," *National Sleep Foundation*, June 15, 2010, www.sleepfoundation.org/article/sleep-topics/shift-work-and-sleep.

15. Caldwell, *Sleep*, 39–40.

16. Ibid., 46.

17. Ibid., 47.

18. Ibid., 27–28.

19. Neubauer, *Understanding Sleeplessness*, 22.

20. Dement, *The Promise of Sleep*, 42.

21. Ibid., 34.

22. Carlos H. Schenck, *Sleep* (New York: Avery, 2007), 32–33.

23. Dement, *The Promise of Sleep*, 19.

24. Dement, *The Promise of Sleep*, 19–20; and Schenck, *Sleep*, 3.

25. Dement, *The Promise of Sleep*, 22–24; and Schenck, *Sleep*, 2–4.

26. Kryger, *A Woman's Guide to Sleep Disorders*, 5–7.

27. Dement, *The Promise of Sleep*, 36–37.

28. Gregory Stores, *Insomnia and Other Adult Sleep Problems* (Oxford and New York: Oxford University Press, 2009), 14.

29. Ibid., 12–13.

30. Dement, *The Promise of Sleep*, 21–22.

31. Schenck, *Sleep*, 5.

Chapter 3

1. Sondra Kornblatt, *Restful Insomnia: How to Get the Benefits of Sleep Even When You Can't* (San Francisco: Wheel/Weiser/LLC, 2010).

2. Ibid.

3. David N. Neubauer, *Understanding Sleeplessness: Perspectives on Insomnia* (Baltimore: The Johns Hopkins University Press, 2003).

Chapter 4

1. T. Berry Brazelton, *TouchPoints: Your Child's Emotional and Behavioral Development* (Menlo Park, CA: Addison-Wesley, 1992), 382–383.

2. Ibid., 384.

3. Elizabeth Pantley, *The No-Cry Sleep Solution: Gentle Ways to Help Your Baby Sleep Through the Night* (New York: McGraw-Hill, 2002).

4. Ibid., xiii–xiv.

5. Stanley Coren, *Sleep Thieves* (New York: Free Press Paperbacks, 1997), 114.

6. Ibid., 114–118.

7. Carlos H. Schenck, *Sleep: A Groundbreaking Guide to the Mysteries, the Problems, and the Solutions* (New York: Avery, 2007), 7.

8. W. C. Dement, *The Promise of Sleep* (New York: Dell, 1999), 105.

9. Coren, *Sleep Thieves*, 106–108.

10. Dement, *The Promise of Sleep*, 399.

11. Gregory Stores, *Insomnia and Other Adult Sleep Problems* (Oxford and New York: Oxford University Press, 2009), 104.

12. L.A. Rosen, "Infant Sleep and Feeding," *Journal of Obstetric, Gynecologic, and Newborn Nursing* 37, no. 6 (2008): 706–714.

13. Brazelton, *TouchPoints*, 388.

14. Rosen, "Infant Sleep and Feeding."

15. Coren, *Sleep Thieves,* 110.

16. "Children and Sleep," *National Sleep Foundation*, Nov 28, 2009, www.sleepfoundation.org/article/sleep-topics/children-and-sleep.

17. Coren, *Sleep Thieves*, 112.

18. Ibid., 113.

19. Dement, *The Promise of Sleep*, 400.

20. Ibid., 401–402.

21. Ibid., 404–406.

22. V. Mark Durand, *When Children*

Don't Sleep Well: Interventions for Pediatric Sleep Disorders Therapist Guide (Oxford: Oxford University Press, 2008), 1–2.

23. Ibid., 5.

24. Ibid., 6.

25. G. Green, *Insomniac* (Los Angeles: University of California Press, 2008), 127–129.

26. Ibid., 121.

27. Durand, *When Children Don't Sleep Well*, 2.

28. "Children and Sleep."

29. Dement, *The Promise of Sleep*, 114.

30. R. Chervin and J. Mindell, "ADHD and Sleep," *National Sleep Foundation*, Nov 28, 2010, www.sleepfoundation.org/article/sleep-topics/adhd-and-sleep.

31. Green, *Insomniac*, 123.

32. Ibid., 124.

33. Ibid., 131.

34. Dement, *The Promise of Sleep*, 114–115.

35. Ibid., 115.

36. Green, *Insomniac*, 159–160.

37. "Sleep and Teens—Biology and Behavior," *National Sleep Foundation*, Nov 28, 2009, www.sleepfoundation.org/article/ask-the-expert/sleep-and-teens-biology-and-behavior. (Article originally appeared in the Spring 2006 issue of *Sleep Matters*.)

38. Dement, *The Promise of Sleep*, 118.

39. Coren, *Sleep Thieves*, 119–120.

40. Dement, *The Promise of Sleep,* 119.

41. John Selby, *Secrets of a Good Night's Sleep* (New York: toExcel, 1999), 44.

42. Dement, *The Promise of Sleep*, 120.

43. Schenck, *Sleep*, 43.

44. M.M. Ohayon, M.A. Carskadon, C. Guilleminauet, and M.V. Vitiella, "Meta-Analysis of Quantitative Sleep Parameters from Childhood to Old Age in Healthy Individuals: Developing Normative Sleep Values Across the Human Lifespan," *Sleep* 27, no. 7 (2004): 1255–1273.

45. J.A. Floyd, J.J. Jamisse, E.S. Jenuwine, and J.W. Ager, "Changes in REM-Sleep Percentage Over the Adult Lifespan," *Sleep* 30, no. 7 (2007): 829–836.

46. M.H. Kryger, *A Woman's Guide to Sleep Disorders* (New York: McGraw-Hill, 2004), 28.

47. Ibid., 35.

48. Ibid., 38.

49. K.A. Lee, G. McEnany, and M.E. Zoffke, "REM Sleep and Mood State in Childbearing Women: Sleepy or Weepy?" *Sleep* 23, no. 7 (2000): 1–9.

50. C. Ruhi, "Sleep Is a Vital Sign: Why Assessing Sleep Is an Important Part of Women's Health," *Nursing for Women's Health* 14, no. 3 (2010): 243–247.

51. Schenck, *Sleep*, 9.

52. "Menopause and Insomnia," *National Sleep Foundation*, Nov 28, 2010, www.sleepfoundation.org/article/ask-the-expert/menopause-and-insomnia.

53. P.A. Minarik, "Sleep Disturbance in Midlife Women," *Journal of Obstetrics, Gynecologic, and Neonatal Nursing* 38, no. 3 (2009): 333–343.

54. E. Van Cauter, R. Leproult, and L. Plat, "Age-Related Changes in Slow Wave Sleep and REM Sleep and Relationship with Growth Hormone and Cortisol Levels in Healthy Men," *The Journal of the American Medical Association* 284, no. 7 (2000): 861–868.

55. David N. Neubauer, *Understanding Sleeplessness: Perspectives on Insomnia* (Baltimore: The Johns Hopkins University Press, 2003), 162.

56. J.R. Espiritu, "Aging-Related Sleep Changes," *Clinical Geriatric Medicine* 24, no. 1 (2008): 1–14.

57. M. Vitiello, "Aging and Sleep," *National Sleep Foundation*, Nov 29, 2010, www.sleepfoundation.org/article/sleep-topics/aging-and-sleep.

58. Selby, *Secrets of a Good Night's Sleep*, 44–45.

59. Neubauer, *Understanding Sleeplessness*, 163–164.

60. Schenck, *Sleep*, 10.

61. Neubauer, *Understanding Sleeplessness*, 164–165.

Chapter 5

1. William Dement, *The Promise of Sleep* (New York: Dell, 1999), 129.

2. Ibid., 130.

3. Gregory Stores, *Insomnia and Other Adult Sleep Problems* (Oxford: Oxford University Press, 2009), 49.

4. Meir H. Kryger, *A Woman's Guide to Sleep Disorders* (New York: McGraw-Hill, 2004), 131.

5. "Delayed Sleep Phase Syndrome," *Wikipedia, the Free Encyclopedia*, http://en.wikipedia.org/wiki/delayed-sleep-phase-syndrome.

6. D. Martinez, M.C. Lenz, and L. Menna-Barreto, "Diagnosis of Circadian Rhythm Sleep Disorders," *Journal of Bras Pneumol* 34, no. 3 (2008): 173–180.

7. "Delayed Sleep Phase Syndrome."

8. N. Zisapel, "Circadian Rhythm Sleep Disorder: Pathophysiology and Potential Approaches to Management," *CNS Drugs* 15, no. 4 (2001): 311–328.

9. Dement, *The Promise of Sleep*, 140–142.

10. Carlos H. Schenck, *Sleep: A Groundbreaking Guide to the Mysteries, the Problems, and the Solutions* (New York: Avery, 2007), 47.

11. Ibid., 51.

12. Gayle Green, *Insomniac* (Berkley: University of California Press, 2008), 356–357.

13. "What Is Restless Legs Syndrome/RLS?" *RLS Foundation and National Sleep Foundation*, www.whatisrls.org/what_is_rls.html ...retrieved 1/28/2010.

14. A. Harding, "Restless Leg Syndrome Runs in Families, Study Confirms," *Reuters*, www.reuters.com/assets/print?aid=USTRE64A4CV20100511.

15. Ibid.

16. "What Is Restless Legs Syndrome/RLS?"

17. Schenck, *Sleep*, 50.

18. S.A. Milligan and A.L. Chesson, "Restless Legs Syndrome in the Older Adult: Diagnosis and Management," *Drugs and Aging* 19, no. 1 (2002): 741–751.

19. "Periodic Limb Movements in Sleep," *National Sleep Foundation*, www.sleepfoundation.org/article/sleep-related-problems/periodic-limb-movements.

20. Schenck, *Sleep*, 52.

21. Stores, *Insomnia and Other Adult Sleep Problems*, 73.

22. "Obstructive Sleep Apnea and Sleep," *National Sleep Foundation*, www.sleepfoundation.org/article/sleep-related-problems/obstructive-sleep-apnea.

23. M. Brogan and V.L. Zeigler, "Obstructive Sleep Apnea: Recognizing an Underdiagnosed Condition," *Clinical Reviews* 20, no. 2 (2010): 24–29.

24. Dement, *The Promise of Sleep*, 182.

25. E. Holohan, "Sleep Apnea Could Raise Heart Risks for Older Men," *Executive Health*, July 12, 2010, www.businessweek.com/lifestyle/content/healthday/641041.html.

26. Kryger, *A Woman's Guide to Sleep Disorders*, 152.

27. Dement, *The Promise of Sleep*, 168.

28. Ibid., 177.

29. "Air Pollution Tied to Breathing Problems in Sleep," *Health Day*, News Release — Brigham and Women's Hospital, http://consumer.healthday.com/article.asp?AID=640140.

30. Brogan and Zeigler, "Obstructive Sleep Apnea."

31. Ibid.

32. Schenck, *Sleep*, 40.

33. Dement, *The Promise of Sleep*, 88–89.

34. Brogan and Zeigler, "Obstructive Sleep Apnea."

35. Dement, *The Promise of Sleep*, 88–89.

36. S.M. Chetlin and C. Landis, "Pain and Sleep: What Is Fibromyalgia?" *National Sleep Foundation*, www.sleepfoundation.org/article/sleep-related-problems/fibromyalgia-nd-sleep.

37. Ibid.

38. Kryger, *A Woman's Guide to Sleep Disorders*, 217.

39. "Depression and Sleep," National Sleep Foundation, www.sleepfoundation.org/article/sleeptopics/depression-and-sleep.

40. Ibid.

Chapter 6

1. David N. Neubauer, *Understanding Sleeplessness: Perspectives on Insomnia* (Baltimore: The Johns Hopkins University Press, 2003).
2. Shere Hite, *The Hite Report: A Nationwide Study of Female Sexuality* (New York: MacMillan, 1976).
3. Neubauer, *Understanding Sleeplessness*, 2–3.
4. Ibid., 10.
5. Ibid. 4.

Chapter 7

1. Michael J. Breus, "Sleep Well," *WebMD*, http://blogs.webmd.com/sleep-disorders/2010/04/is-sexsomnia-real.html.
2. R.H. Epstein, "Raiding the Refrigerator, but Still Asleep," *The New York Times Health*, April 7, 2010, http://nytimes.com/2010/04/07eating.html?ref=health.
3. D. Tuncel, "Parasomnias: Diagnosis, Classification and Clinical Features," *Psikiyatride Guncel Yaklasemlar* 1, no. 3 (2009): 280–296.
4. William C. Dement, *The Promise of Sleep* (New York: Dell, 1999), 195.
5. Gregory Stores, *Insomnia and Other Adult Health Problems* (Oxford: Oxford University Press, 2009), 87.
6. Carlos H. Schenck, *Sleep: A Groundbreaking Guide to the Mysteries, the Problems, and the Solutions* (New York: Avery, 2007), 66.
7. Ibid., 68.
8. M. Mahowald, "Sleep Walking," *National Sleep Foundation*, www.sleepfoundation.org/article/sleep-related-problems/sleepwalking.
9. Schenck, *Sleep*, 100–102.
10. Dement, *The Promise of Sleep*, 211–214.
11. Schenck, *Sleep*, 103.
12. Ibid., 104.
13. Ibid., 108, 111.
14. Meir H. Kryger, *A Woman's Guide to Sleep Disorders* (New York: McGraw-Hill 2004), 197.
15. Dement, *The Promise of Sleep*, 211.

16. Schenck, *Sleep*, 144–149.
17. Ibid., 156.
18. Stores, *Insomnia and Other Adult Health Problems*, 96.
19. Dement, *The Promise of Sleep*, 457.
20. Epstein, "Raiding the Refrigerator, but Still Asleep."
21. Schenck, *Sleep*, 183–185.
22. Ibid., 186–187.
23. Ibid., 129–132.
24. Breus, "Sleep Well."
25. Schenck, *Sleep*, 140–141.
26. David N. Neubauer, *Understanding Sleeplessness: Perspectives on Insomnia* (Baltimore: The Johns Hopkins Press, 2003), 134–135.
27. Stores, *Insomnia and Other Adult Health Problems*, 92.
28. _____. "REM Behavior Disorder and Sleep," *National Sleep Foundation*, www.sleepfoundation.org/article/sleep-related-problems/rem-behavior-disorder-and.
29. Kryger, *A Woman's Guide to Sleep Disorders*, 194–195.
30. Dement, *The Promise of Sleep*, 208–209.
31. _____. "REM Behavior Disorder and Sleep."
32. Schenck, *Sleep*, 230–231.
33. _____. "Narcolepsy," *Healthline*, www.healthline.com?adamcontent/narcolepsy?utm_source=narcolepsy&utm_ad=wh.
34. Stores, *Insomnia*, 77.
35. Ibid.
36. Dement, *The Promise of Sleep*, 197.
37. Ibid., 200–201.
38. _____, "Narcolepsy," *Healthline*.
39. D. T. Max, *The Family That Couldn't Sleep* (New York: Random House, 2006).
40. Ibid., xiv–xv.
41. D. T. Max, "The Secrets of Sleep," *National Geographic* (May 2010): 76.
42. Max, *The Family That Couldn't Sleep*, 19.

Chapter 8

1. David N. Neubauer, *Understanding Sleeplessness: Perspectives on Insomnia*

(Baltimore: The Johns Hopkins Press, 2003), 14.

2. Stanley Coren, *Sleep Thieves* (New York: Free Press Paperbacks, 1996), 169–173.

3. _____. "One Sleepless Night Ups Insulin Resistance," *Health Day*. The Endocrine Society News Release, May 5, 2010, www.healthday.com/Article.asp?AID=638788.

4. D.T. Max, "The Secrets of Sleep," *National Geographic* (May 2010): 80.

5. Neubauer, *Understanding Sleeplessness*, 11–12.

6. Carlos H. Schenck, *Sleep: A Groundbreaking Guide to the Mysteries, the Problems, and the Solutions* (New York: Avery, 2007), 11.

7. Meir H. Kryger, *A Woman's Guide to Sleep Disorders* (New York: McGraw-Hill, 2004), 108.

8. A. Norton, "Sleep Problems Linked to Weight Gain in Middle Age," *Reuters*, www.reuters.com/article/idUSTRE6612/RD20100702.

9. Max, "The Secrets of Sleep," 91.

10. Ibid., 80–82.

11. William C. Dement, *The Promise of Sleep* (New York: Dell, 1999), 225.

12. Max, "The Secrets of Sleep," 80–82.

13. Coren, *Sleep Thieves*, 238.

14. Max, "The Secrets of Sleep," 90.

15. Dement, *The Promise of Sleep*, 226–227.

16. Max, "The Secrets of Sleep," 81.

Chapter 9

1. William C. Dement, *The Promise of Sleep* (New York: Dell, 1999), 150.

2. Michael Breus, "Sleep Well," *WebMD*, http://blogs.webmd.com/sleep-disorders/2010/05/regular-daily-routines-enhance-sleep-exp.

3. D. T. Max, "The Secrets of Sleep," *National Geographic* (May 2010): 81.

4. _____. *Mosby's Nursing Drug Reference*, 22nd ed. (St. Louis, MO: Mosby, 2009), 70.

5. J. Paul Caldwell, *Sleep: A Complete Guide to Sleep Disorders and a Better Night's Sleep* (Buffalo, NY: Firefly Books, 2003), 228–229.

6. Ibid., 229.

7. Ibid., 232–233.

8. Gregory Stores, *Insomnia and Other Adult Sleep Problems* (Oxford: Oxford University Press, 2009), 55.

9. Ibid., 56.

10. Dement, *The Promise of Sleep*, 157.

11. David N. Neubauer, "Current and New Thinking in the Management of Comorbid Insomnia," *American Journal of Managed Care* 15 (Feb. 2009): S24–32.

12. Caldwell, *Sleep*, 218–219.

13. Dement, *The Promise of Sleep*, 154–155.

14. Caldwell, *Sleep*, 223–224.

15. Dement, *The Promise of Sleep*, 152.

16. David N. Neubauer, Understanding Sleeplessness: Perspectives on Insomnia (Baltimore: The Johns Hopkins Press, 2003), 95.

17. Ibid., 112.

18. Ibid., 107–108.

19. Ibid., 110.

20. Ibid., 110–111.

21. Max, "Secrets of Sleep," 86–87.

22. L. Lyon, "Battling Insomnia? Consider Therapy," *U.S. News & World Report* (Dec. 2009): 76–77.

23. C.M. Morin, R.R. Bootzin, D.J. Buysse, J.D. Edinger, C.A. Espie, and K.L. Lichstein, "Psychological and Behavioral Treatment of Insomnia: Update of the Recent Evidence (1998–2004)," *Sleep* 29, no. 11 (2006): 1398–1414.

24. Sondra Kornblatt, *Restful Insomnia* (San Francisco: Red Wheel/Weiser, LLC, 2010), 42.

25. Ibid. 43, 52–53.

Chapter 10

1. David N. Neubauer, *Understanding Sleeplessness: Perspectives on Insomnia* (Baltimore: The Johns Hopkins University Press, 2003), 2–3.

2. Ibid.

3. Ibid., 2.

4. S. Ancoli-Israel and T. Roth, "Char-

acteristics of Insomnia in the United States: Results of the 1991 National Sleep Foundation Survey," *Sleep* 22 (suppl 2): S347–53; as reported in Neubauer, *op.cit.*, 10.

5. Neubauer, *op.cit.*, 10.

6. F.J. Zorick and J.K. Walsh, "Evaluation and Management of Insomnia: An Overview," in *Principles and Practice of Sleep Medicine*, 3d ed., edited by Meir H. Kryger, T. Roth, and William C. Dement (Philadelphia: W.B. Saunders: 615–623); as reported in Neubauer, *op.cit.*, 10–11.

7. Sondra Kornblatt, *Restful Insomnia* (San Francisco: Red Wheel/Weiser, LLC, 2010).

8. Neubauer, *op. cit.*

Chapter 11

1. John Selby, *Secrets of a Good Night's Sleep* (New York: toExcel, 1999), 15–16.

2. *Carl Jung: Dreams and Philosophy* (Filiquarian, 2008), available for download at www.biographiq.com/bookd/CJDP458.

Selected Bibliography

Brazelton, T.B. *TouchPoints: Your Child's Emotional and Behavioral Development*. Mento Park, CA: Addison-Wesley, 1992.

Caldwell, J.P. *Sleep: A Complete Guide to Sleep Disorders and a Better Night's Sleep*. Buffalo: Firefly Books, 2003.

Coren, S. *Sleep Thieves*. New York: Free Press Paperbacks, 1996.

Dement, W. *The Promise of Sleep*. New York: Dell, 1999.

Durand, V.M. *When Children Don't Sleep Well: Interventions for Pediatric Sleep Disorders Therapist Guide*. Oxford: Oxford University Press, 2008.

Green, G. *Insomniac*. Berkeley: University of California Press, 2008.

Kornblatt, S. *Restful Insomnia*. San Francisco: Red Wheel/Weiser, 2010.

Kryger, M.H. *A Woman's Guide to Sleep Disorders*. New York: McGraw-Hill, 2004.

Max, D.T. *The Family That Couldn't Sleep*. New York: Random House, 2006.

Neubauer, D.N. *Understanding Sleeplessness: Perspectives on Insomnia*. Baltimore: The Johns Hopkins University Press, 2003.

Pantley, E. *The No-Cry Sleep Solution: Gentle Ways to Help Your Baby Sleep Through the Night*. New York: McGraw-Hill, 2002.

Schenck, C.H. *Sleep: A Groundbreaking Guide to the Mysteries, the Problems, and the Solutions* . New York: Avery, 2007.

Selby, J. *Secrets of a Good Night's Sleep*. New York: toExcel, 1999.

Stores, G. *Insomnia and Other Adult Sleep Problems*. Oxford and New York: Oxford University Press, 2009.

About the Authors

Phyllis Levin Brodsky, RNC, MS, received her initial nurse training immediately after high school in the former three-year, in-house, training program of the Albert Einstein Medical Center of Philadelphia, in 1954 to 1957. After a number of hospital positions, centering in the main on obstetric and gynecological services, she returned to studies at the University of Maryland, where she completed a B.S. and M.S. in nursing education. After that, she held teaching positions in several colleges and universities, became certified in obstetric and gynecological nursing as well as in childbirth education, and continued various professional pursuits in lecturing and community services. In addition to publishing several articles in nursing journals, she authored two books published in 2008: *Women in Childbirth: Women vs. Medicine Through the Ages* (McFarland); and *Memoirs of a Student Nurse, or "You can leave any time you want"* (Cats Paw Publications).

Allen Brodsky, Sc.D., CHP, CIH, DABR, has been an adjunct professor at Georgetown University since 1987. His education includes a B.E. in 1949 in chemical engineering at Johns Hopkins University; a one-year Atomic Energy Commission–National Research Council fellowship in radiological physics in 1949-1950 at Oak Ridge National Laboratory; a master's degree in physics in 1960 at Johns Hopkins; and a doctor of science in hygiene in 1966 at the Graduate School of Public Health, University of Pittsburgh. He has reviewed research proposals for five Federal agencies, has published original statistical methods, and has written chapters on statistical methods in the second of his four-volume *Handbook of Radiation Measurement and Protection* (CRC Press, 1979–1986). Other publications include the book *Review of Radiation Risks and Uranium Toxicity* (RSA Publications, Hebron, CT, 1996); the edited volume (in which he was also the author of several chapters) *Public Protection from Nuclear, Chemical, and Biological Terrorism* (Medical Physics Publishing, Madison, WI, 2004); and many journal articles and reports. He received the Distinguished Graduate Award of the University of Pittsburgh Graduate School of Public Health in 2004, "in recognition of his outstanding contributions to the field of public health."

Index